Discover the secrets and techniques of the Mediterranean diet And Veganism with the

Green Plate Diet

: Expert Advice and Over 4 hundred Delicious Easy-to-Follow Recipes

O'Christ. O

TABLE OF CONTENT

Introduction:

Chapter 1: Introduction

- Brief overview of the Mediterranean diet and veganism
- Benefits of transitioning to a plant-based diet

Chapter 2: The Mediterranean Diet

- History and origins of the Mediterranean diet
- Key components of the diet
- Health benefits of the Mediterranean diet

Chapter 3: Veganism

- History and origins of veganism
- Key components of a vegan diet
- Health benefits of veganism

Chapter 4: The Science of Nutrition

- Overview of nutrition science
- Nutritional requirements for a healthy diet
- How to get all the nutrients you need on a plant-based diet

Chapter 5: Getting Started

- Tips for transitioning to a plant-based diet
- How to stock your pantry and fridge
- Meal planning and preparation

Chapter 6: Breakfast Recipes

- Delicious and healthy breakfast recipes

Chapter 7: Lunch Recipes

- Delicious and healthy lunch recipes

Chapter 8: Dinner Recipes

- Delicious and healthy dinner recipes

Chapter 9: Snacks and Desserts

- Healthy and satisfying snack and dessert recipes

Chapter 10: Staying Motivated

- Tips for staying motivated on your plant-based journey
- Common challenges and how to overcome them

Introduction

Are you equipped to take your health to the subsequent degree? Don't search any further than "Discover the secrets and techniques of the Mediterranean diet and Veganism with the Green Plate Diet: Expert Advice and Over 4 hundred Delicious Easy-to-Follow Recipes". This complete guide is filled with the modern-day research and insights on of the world's maximum famous diets. With direct and tasty language, you'll discover the secrets and techniques and strategies of the Mediterranean Diet and Veganism, and discover ways to rework your fitness with over four hundred scrumptious and clean-to-observe recipes. Whether you're a pro vegan or simply beginning out, this book has the entirety you want to enjoy wholesome and gratifying food so as to leave you feeling energized and refreshed. Whether you want to lose weight or stay motivated overall. Whether you want to improve your physical health or just feel better, this book is the perfect guide to achieving your goals.

Research shows these diets can help reduce the risk of chronic diseases such as heart disease, diabetes, and cancer. In particular, the Mediterranean diet is associated with a longer lifespan and lower risk of Alzheimer's disease. Veganism is now proven to help you lose weight, lower blood sugar levels, and improve kidney function. Combining the best of both worlds, "Discover the secrets and techniques of the Mediterranean diet and Veganism with the Green Plate Diet: Expert Advice and Over 4 hundred Delicious Easy-to-Follow Recipes" provides a comprehensive and effective approach to healthy eating.

Utilizing the latest nutrition science, this book is the ultimate guide to transitioning to a healthier, plant-based lifestyle. So why wait? Start your adventure to better health today with The Green Plate Diet

CHAPTER 1: INTRODUCTION TO THE MEDITERRANEAN DIET AND VEGANISM

"Are you interested in improving your overall health and well-being?? Do you want to make a positive change in your life but don't know where to start? Look no further than the Mediterranean diet and veganism. These two dietary patterns have been shown to offer a wide range of health benefits, from reducing the risk of chronic diseases to improving overall quality of life.

The Mediterranean diet is based on the traditional dietary habits of people living in countries surrounding the Mediterranean Sea. It promotes the consumption of whole, minimally processed foods such as fruits, vegetables, whole grains, legumes, nuts, seeds, and olive oil. Studies have shown that the Mediterranean diet helps to reduce the risk of heart disease, stroke, and other chronic conditions.

Meanwhile, veganism is a dietary pattern that excludes all animal products, including meat, dairy, and eggs. Veganism has been shown to help with weight loss, lower blood sugar levels, and improve kidney function.

By combining the best of both worlds, the Mediterranean diet and veganism offer a comprehensive and effective approach to healthy eating. With the latest updates on nutrition science, this book is the ultimate guide to transitioning to a healthier, plant-based lifestyle."

• Overview of the Mediterranean Diet and Veganism

A Brief Overview of the Mediterranean Diet and Veganism

The Mediterranean Diet and veganism are two popular diets that are being studied for their health benefits.

The Mediterranean diet is based on traditional foods eaten in countries such as Italy and Greece in the 1960s. Focus on minimally processed, whole foods and limit or avoid animal products. On the other hand, is a lifestyle aimed at eliminating the use of animals for food, clothing, and other purposes.

It is a completely plant-based diet, avoiding all animal products and dairy products such as cheese, yogurt, and eggs, and consuming only plant-based foods.

According to a study published in the Journal of Internal Medicine, the Mediterranean diet is associated with numerous health benefits. It is associated with a lower risk of chronic diseases such as heart disease, cancer, and diabetes.

This is because the Mediterranean diet is rich in fiber, vitamins, minerals, and antioxidants that are essential for good health. The Mediterranean diet also emphasizes healthy fats, such as olive oil, and limits red meat and processed foods.

Vegetarianism is also associated with a lower risk of chronic disease.

A study published in the Journal of the American Heart Association found that a plant-based diet is associated with a lower risk of heart disease.

This is because plant-based diets are naturally low in saturated fat and high in fiber, which can help lower cholesterol and improve heart health.

Veganism also has environmental benefits, reducing the demand for animal products that contribute to greenhouse gas emissions and deforestation.

There are some similarities between the Mediterranean diet and veganism.

Both diets are primarily based on plant-based foods, and in fact he can combine the two diets with a vegan Mediterranean diet that follows the basic principles of both diets. However, the Mediterranean diet leaves more room for animal products, with an emphasis on fatty fish, lean meat, and eggs rather than red meat.

A vegan diet is completely plant-based, and many vegans take supplements to provide certain nutrients that they may be lacking because they don't eat animal products.

Both the Mediterranean diet and veganism are associated with numerous health benefits.

The Mediterranean diet emphasizes minimally processed, whole foods and limits or avoids animal products, while veganism is a completely plant-based diet that avoids all animal products and dairy products. Both diets are primarily based on plant-based foods, and in fact he can combine the two diets with a vegan Mediterranean diet that follows the basic principles of both diets.

• **Advantages of Embracing a Plant-Based Diet**

A plant-based diet is one that emphasizes minimally processed, whole foods and limits or eliminates animal products.

A proponent of a plant-based diet, focusing on whole foods from plant sources can reduce weight, blood pressure, and risk of heart disease, cancer, and diabetes.

Here are some of The Advantages of Embracing a Plant-Based Diet:

1. **Lower risk of chronic diseases**: Plant-based diets are associated with lower risks of chronic diseases such as heart disease, cancer, and diabetes. This is because plant-based diets are rich in fiber, vitamins, minerals, and antioxidants that are essential for good health.

2. **Improved Gut Health**: A plant-based diet improves your gut health, allowing you to better absorb nutrients from foods that support your immune system and reduce inflammation.

3. **Environmental Sustainability**: Globally, the meat industry has a significant impact on water, soil, extinction of plants and animals, consumption of natural resources, and contributes significantly to global warming.

4. **Weight Management**: Plant-based diets are naturally low in calories and high in fiber, which can help you maintain a healthy weight.

5. **Reduced risk of certain cancers**: studies suggest that a plant-based diet is associated with a reduced risk of certain cancers.

6. **Improved Athletic Performance**: A plant-based diet can improve athletic performance by providing the nutrients needed for optimal muscle function and recovery.

7. **Cost-effective**: Plant-based diets can be more cost-effective than meat and dairy diets.

CHAPTER 2: THE MEDITERRANEAN DIET

· History and Origins of the Mediterranean Diet

The Mediterranean Diet is a social practice based on a set of skills, knowledge, customs, and traditions, from landscape to cuisine.

Countries of Mediterranean culture are concerned with cultivation, harvesting, fishing, preservation, processing, preparation, and especially consumption.

This diet is characterized by a high intake of plant-based foods, such as fruits, vegetables, whole grains, legumes, and nuts, and a low intake of animal-based foods, such as red meat and dairy products.

The Mediterranean diet is rich in healthy fats, especially olive oil, and also includes fish and poultry in moderation. The Mediterranean diet has its roots in the Mediterranean region, which includes her 22 countries in Europe, Africa, and Asia.

The origins of nutrition reflect the interactions of different populations and civilizations over thousands of years. The concept of the Mediterranean diet was developed in the 1960s to reflect the dietary patterns typical of Crete, most of Greece, and Italy.

This diet was first published in 1975 by American biologist Ansel Keys and his wife, chemist Margaret Keys.

Since then, the Mediterranean diet has become widely known for having some of the lowest health benefits in the world, including lower mortality rates from cardiovascular disease and some types of cancer, as well as lower rates of chronic disease overall.

The Mediterranean diet has evolved over time due to globalization and technological advances, resulting in changes to the traditional diet.

Nevertheless, nutrition continues to be a topic of great research interest.

Since 1993, diet, nutrition, and health experts have held a series of conferences to discuss research on the composition and health effects of the Mediterranean diet.

The result is the Mediterranean Diet Guide Pyramid, which encourages healthy food choices.

• Main Elements of the Diet

The Mediterranean diet is a healthy eating pattern that emphasizes the intake of plant-based foods, healthy fats, and lean protein sources.

According to the American Heart Association, the main ingredients of the Mediterranean diet are:

• Vegetables

• Fruits

• Whole grains

• Legumes

• Nuts and seeds

• Olive oil

• Seafood

• Poultry

• Dairy products (cheese and yogurt)

• Moderate alcohol intake (Mainly wine with meals)

• **Vegetables**: An essential component of the Mediterranean diet is vegetables..

Rich in vitamins, minerals and fiber. Examples of vegetables include tomatoes, cucumbers, eggplants, zucchini, and peppers.

• **Fruits**: Fruits are another important part of the Mediterranean diet. It offers an abundance of vitamins, minerals, and fiber.. Examples of fruits include oranges, apples, grapes, and pomegranates.

• **Whole grains**: Vitamins, minerals, and fiber are found in whole grains.It's also low in fat. Examples of whole grains include brown rice, quinoa, whole grain bread, and whole grain pasta.

• **Legumes**: Legumes are an excellent source of protein, fiber, and minerals. It's also low in fat. Examples of legumes include chickpeas, lentils, and beans.

• **Nuts and Seeds**: Healthy fats, protein, and fiber can be obtained from nuts and seeds. Examples of nuts and seeds include almonds, walnuts, pistachios, and chia seeds.

• **Olive oil**: Olive oil is a staple of the Mediterranean diet. Rich in healthy fats and antioxidants. It is used as a salad dressing, cooking oil, and bread dip.

• **Seafood**: Seafood is a good source of protein and healthy fats. It also contains almost no saturated fat. Examples of seafood include salmon, tuna, sardines, and shrimp.

• **Chicken**: Chicken is a good source of protein and is lower in fat than red meat. Examples of poultry include chickens and turkeys.

• **Dairy products (cheese and yogurt)**: Dairy products are a good source of calcium and protein. Examples of dairy products include feta cheese, Greek yogurt, and kefir.

• **Moderate alcohol intake (mainly wine with meals)**: Moderate alcohol intake is part of the Mediterranean diet. Red wine is the preferred choice. It is rich in antioxidants and has been associated with a reduced risk of heart disease.

The Mediterranean diet is not a restrictive diet, but a lifestyle that promotes healthy eating habits. Associated with reduced risk of heart disease, high blood pressure, and other chronic diseases.

• **Healthy Advantages of the Mediterranean Diet**

The Mediterranean Diet is a healthy diet that has been around for a very long time. The emphasis is on eating plant-based foods, healthy fats, and lean protein sources. It was chosen as the best overall diet, best for healthy eating, easiest to implement, and best plant-based diet.

Studies show that adherence to a Mediterranean diet is associated with a lower risk of developing cardiovascular disease, type 2 diabetes, respiratory diseases such as chronic obstructive pulmonary disease, including neurodegenerative diseases like Alzheimer's and Parkinson's. The Mediterranean diet is also associated with lower risk of heart disease, improved brain and gut health, and lower risk of cancer.

The Mediterranean diet is not a dietary restriction, but a lifestyle that promotes healthy eating habits. The focus is on minimally processed, whole foods, and placing primarily plants on your plate rather than red meat.

You can follow a Mediterranean eating pattern by making a few simple changes to your shopping list.

• Make vegetables the center of your cooking. Eat less meat and add more vegetables to your plate.

• Avoid meat at least once a week.

• Cook more meals with beans.

• Enjoy seafood twice a week. Fatty fish such as salmon, mackerel, and sardines are good for your heart and brain.

• Eat dairy products. Enjoy plain Greek yogurt and a little cheese.

• Switch to whole grains.

Avoid refined white grains and opt for barley, brown rice, and oats.

• Add fresh fruit.

You can eat it as a snack or enjoy it as a dessert.

Research shows that adherence to a Mediterranean diet is associated with a lower risk of developing cardiovascular disease, type 2 diabetes, respiratory diseases such as chronic obstructive pulmonary disease.

The Mediterranean diet is rich in fruits, vegetables, legumes, whole grains, and nuts, which are rich in antioxidants, vitamins, minerals, and fiber. These foods are associated with reduced inflammation, improved immune function, and lower risk of chronic disease.

CHAPTER 3: VEGANISM

· History and Origins of Veganism

Veganism is a philosophy and way of life aimed at eliminating all forms of exploitation and animal cruelty for any purpose. It also encourages the development of cruelty-free alternatives and products.

Veganism is a lifestyle that avoids the use of animal products, including food, clothing, and other items. Vegans avoid meat, dairy products, eggs, and honey, as well as products that have been tested on animals or are made with animal-derived ingredients.

· Key elements of a vegan diet that's right!

A vegan diet is a plant-based diet that excludes all animal products such as meat, dairy, eggs, and honey.

It is important that a vegan diet is balanced and ensures that it provides all the nutrients necessary for good health.

Here are some important components of a vegan diet:

1. **Fruits and vegetables**: These are an essential part of a vegan diet and provide a wide range of vitamins, minerals, and antioxidants.

2. **Whole grains**: Whole grain products such as brown rice, quinoa, and whole grain bread are rich in fiber, vitamins, and minerals.

3. **Legumes**: Legumes such as beans, lentils, and chickpeas are good sources of protein, fiber, and iron.

4. **Nuts and Seeds**: Nuts and seeds are an excellent source of healthy fats, protein, and fiber. It is also rich in vitamins and minerals such as vitamin E, magnesium, and zinc.

5. **Fortified Foods**: Vegans need to get enough vitamin B12,

vitamin D, and calcium, which are essential for good health. You can get these nutrients from fortified foods such as plant-based milks, breakfast cereals, and nutritional yeast.

6. **Plant-based milks**: Plant-based milks such as soy milk, almond milk, and oat milk are good sources of calcium and vitamin D. It is also low in fat and calories, making it an ideal substitute for milk.

7. **Plant-based protein sources**: Vegans need to eat enough protein, which is essential for building and repairing tissues in the body. Good sources of plant-based protein include tofu, tempeh, and seitan.

8. **Healthy Fats**: Healthy fats, found in foods such as avocados, nuts, and seeds, are important for good health. These help reduce inflammation in the body and lower the risk of heart disease.

In summary, a vegan diet should include a variety of fruits, vegetables, whole grains, legumes, nuts, and seeds. Fortified foods and plant-based milks provide important nutrients such as vitamin B12, vitamin D, and calcium.

Plant-based protein sources and healthy fats are also important components of a vegan diet.

• **Health Benefits of Veganism**

Veganism is a lifestyle that has become increasingly popular in recent years. According to the BBC article, veganism is generally higher in fiber and lower in cholesterol, protein, calcium, and salt than omnivorous diets.

The health benefits of veganism are:

1. **Weight Loss**: A vegan diet helps you lose weight. Several randomized controlled trials have reported that vegan diets are more effective for weight loss than other diets. Vegan meals generally contain more fiber, which can help you feel fuller and reduce your calorie intake.

2. **Reduced risk of heart disease**: A vegan diet can help reduce your risk of heart disease by lowering your cholesterol levels. A study of 48,000 people over the age of 18 found that those who followed a vegan and vegetarian diet had a lower risk of heart

disease than those who ate meat,

3. **Reduced risk of diabetes**: A vegan diet lowers blood sugar levels and reduces the risk of type 2 diabetes. A vegan diet also offers some protection against type 2 diabetes and certain cancers.

4. **Improving kidney function**: A vegan diet can help improve kidney function in people with kidney disease. A plant-based diet is also associated with a lower risk of chronic kidney disease.

5. **Arthritis Pain Relief**: A vegan diet can help reduce inflammation in the body and relieve arthritis pain. A vegan diet is rich in antioxidants and anti-inflammatory compounds that help reduce inflammation in the body.

6. **Improves gut health**: A vegan diet is rich in fiber, which helps improve gut health by promoting the growth of healthy gut bacteria. A healthy gut microbiome is associated with a lower risk of chronic diseases such as heart disease, diabetes, and cancer.

7. **Anti-inflammatory**: A vegan diet is rich in antioxidants and anti-inflammatory compounds that help reduce inflammation in the body. Chronic inflammation is associated with increased risk of chronic diseases such as heart disease, diabetes, and cancer.

Veganism offers several health benefits, including weight loss, reduced risk of heart disease and diabetes, improved kidney function, reduced arthritis pain, improved gut health, and anti-inflammatory effects.

CHAPTER 4: THE SCIENCE OF NUTRITION

Nutrition is the study of how food affects the body and how the body uses food.

This includes all aspects of food, from how it is ingested to how it is metabolized in the body.

• Introduction to Nutritional Science

Nutrition is the intake of nutritional substances that enable living organisms to grow, maintain, and reproduce.

Nutritional science is constantly evolving and new research is being conducted all the time. For example, a recent study found that a ketogenic diet may be effective in controlling polycystic kidney disease.

Another study found that certain human genetic variants in a receptor that stimulates insulin secretion may make people more resistant to obesity.

Maintaining good health and preventing chronic diseases relies on nutrition. For example, a vegan diet offers several health benefits, including weight loss, reduced risk of heart disease and diabetes, improved kidney function, reduced arthritis pain, improved gut health, and anti-inflammatory effects.

It has been shown that A balanced vegan diet should include a variety of fruits, vegetables, whole grains, legumes, nuts, and seeds. Fortified foods and plant-based milks provide important nutrients such as vitamin B12, vitamin D, and calcium. Plant-based protein sources and healthy fats are also important components of a vegan diet.

• **Essential nutrients for a healthy diet.**

A healthy diet is essential for good health and helps prevent chronic diseases such as heart disease, stroke, and diabetes. According to the World Health Organization (WHO), a healthy diet should include a variety of fruits, vegetables, legumes, nuts, and whole grains. It is recommended to consume at least 5 servings of fruits and vegetables daily, excluding potatoes, sweet potatoes, cassava, and other starchy roots. WHO also recommends limiting free sugar intake to less than 10% of total energy intake and salt intake to less than 5g per day? Energy intake (calories) must be balanced with energy expenditure, and total fat content should not exceed 30% of total energy intake. Saturated fat intake should be less than 10% of total energy intake, Trans fat intake should be less than 1% of total energy intake, and fat consumption should shift from saturated and trans fats to unsaturated fats.

A healthy diet should also include a variety of protein sources, such as seafood, lean meats and poultry, eggs, legumes, soy products, nuts and seeds.

Note that the exact composition of a diverse, balanced, and healthy diet will vary depending on individual characteristics such as age, gender, lifestyle, and level of physical activity, as well as cultural background and locally available foods.

• **How to Get All the Nutrients You Need on a Plant-Based Diet**

A plant-based diet, if balanced and varied, can provide you with all the nutrients you need for good health. A healthy vegan diet includes at least five servings of a variety of fruits and vegetables each day, with a base of potatoes, bread, rice, pasta, or other starchy carbohydrates (preferably whole grains). Consume beans, legumes, and other proteins such as soy drinks and yogurt (choose low-fat and low-sugar options), eat nuts and seeds daily that are rich in omega-3 fatty acids (such as walnuts), and choose unsaturated oils. eat small portions with spreads, consume fortified foods and supplements that contain nutrients that are difficult to obtain from a vegan diet, such as vitamin D, vitamin B12, iodine, selenium, calcium, and iron, and drink plenty of water.

It is important that a vegan diet is balanced and ensures that it provides all the nutrients necessary for good health.

Here are some important components of a vegan diet:

1. **Fruits and vegetables**: These are an essential part of a vegan diet and provide a wide range of vitamins, minerals, and antioxidants. We recommend consuming at least 5 servings of fruits and vegetables daily.

2. **Whole grains**: Brown rice, quinoa, and whole-wheat bread are examples of whole grains that are high in fiber, vitamins, and minerals. Additionally, it serves as a beneficial source of energy-providing carbohydrates.

3. **Legumes**: Legumes such as beans, lentils, and chickpeas are good sources of protein, fiber, and iron. Additionally, it has low fat and calorie content, making it an ideal food for weight loss.

4. **Nuts and Seeds**: Nuts and seeds are an excellent source of healthy fats, protein, and fiber. It is also rich in vitamins and minerals such as vitamin E, magnesium, and zinc.

5. **Fortified Foods**: Vegans need to get enough vitamin B12, vitamin D, and calcium, which are essential for good health. You can get these nutrients from fortified foods such as plant-based milks, breakfast cereals, and nutritional yeast.

6. **Plant-based milks**: Plant-based milks such as soy milk, almond milk, and oat milk are good sources of calcium and vitamin D. It is also low in fat and calories, making it an ideal substitute for milk.

7. **Plant-based protein sources**: Vegans need to consume enough protein, which is essential for building and repairing tissues in the body. Good sources of plant-based protein include tofu, tempeh, and seitan.

8. **Healthy Fats**: Healthy fats, found in foods such as avocados,

nuts, and seeds, are important for good health. These help reduce inflammation in the body and lower the risk of heart disease.

In summary, a vegan diet should include a variety of fruits, vegetables, whole grains, legumes, nuts, and seeds. Fortified foods and plant-based milks provide important nutrients such as vitamin B12, vitamin D, and calcium. Plant-based protein sources and healthy fats are also important components of a vegan diet.

CHAPTER 5: GETTING STARTED

· Tips for Switching to a Plant-Based Diet

Switching to a plant-based diet can be difficult, but it's definitely worth it.

1. **Start slow**: When transitioning to a plant-based diet, it's important to take your time. Start by incorporating more plant-based foods into your diet and gradually reduce your intake of animal products.

2. **Focus on whole foods**: Whole foods, such as fruits, vegetables, whole grains, and legumes, should be the basis of your diet. These foods are packed with nutrients and will leave you feeling full and satisfied.

3. **Find plant-based alternatives**: There are many plant-based alternatives to animal products such as meat, dairy, and eggs. Experiment with different plant-based milks, cheeses, and meat substitutes to find what works best for you.

4. **Plan your meals**: Planning your meals in advance can help you stay on track with a plant-based diet. Make a shopping list and plan next week's meals.

5. **Get Support**: It may be helpful to get support from others who are also switching to a plant-based diet. Join a local vegan or vegetarian group.

6. **Get educated**: Stay motivated and engaged by learning about the benefits of a plant-based diet.

7. **Be patient**: Switching to a plant-based diet is a process and it's important to be patient with you.

Don't beat yourself up if you fail or make a mistake.

Just keep moving forward and focus on the positive changes you are making.

• **How to Stock Your Pantry and Refrigerator** stocking your pantry and refrigerator with vegan foods is easy and affordable.

1. **Grains**: Stock up on whole grains like brown rice, quinoa, and whole-wheat pasta. These are versatile ingredients that can be used in a variety of dishes.

2. **Canned**: Canned beans, lentils, and chickpeas are an excellent source of protein and can be used in soups, stews, and salads. Canned tomatoes are also a versatile ingredient that can be used in a variety of dishes.

3. **Nuts and Seeds**: Nuts and seeds are an excellent source of healthy fats, protein, and fiber. Stock up on almonds, cashews, walnuts, chia seeds, and flaxseeds.

4. **Plant-based milks**: Plant-based milks such as soy milk, almond milk, and oat milk are excellent alternatives to cow's milk. Can be used in smoothies, cereal, baking, etc.

5. **Fresh Food**: Stock up on fresh fruits and vegetables, such as leafy greens, carrots, cucumbers, and berries. These are essential ingredients for a healthy vegan diet.

6. **Tofu and Tempeh**: Tofu and tempeh are excellent sources of protein and can be used in a variety of dishes. It can be marinated, grilled, or sautéed.

7. **Herbs and Spices**: Herbs and spices are essential for adding flavor to vegan dishes. Stock up on basil, oregano, thyme, cumin, and chili powder.

8. **Nutritional Yeast**: Nutritional yeast is an excellent source of vitamin B12 and can be used to add cheesy flavor to vegan dishes.

9. **Frozen Fruits and Vegetables**: Frozen fruits and vegetables are a great way to stock up on out-of-season produce. Can be used in smoothies, stir-fries, and soups.

10. **Vegan condiments**: Stock up on vegan condiments like mustard, ketchup, and hot sauce. These can be used to add flavor to sandwiches, burgers, and salads. Stocking your pantry and

fridge with vegan foods is easy and affordable.

Grains, canned foods, nuts and seeds, plant-based milks, fresh produce, tofu and tempeh, herbs and spices, nutritional yeast, frozen fruits and vegetables, and vegan spices are all essential ingredients for a healthy vegan diet.

• Meal Planning and Preparation Meal planning and preparation is a great way to stay on track with your vegan diet.

1. **Plan your meals**: Planning your meals in advance will help you stay on track with your vegan diet. Make a shopping list and plan next week's meals.

2. **Stock up on essentials**: Whole grains, canned beans, nuts and seeds, non-dairy milk, fresh produce, tofu and tempeh, herbs and spices, nutritional yeast, frozen fruit, vegetables and vegan spices.

3. **Meal Prep**: Preparing meals in advance can save you time throughout the week. Cook up a pot of beans and whole grains every week. Grill one or two vegetables.

Please prepare your favorite salad dressings and sauces. Wash and prepare the lettuce.

4. **Get creative**: Experiment with different plant-based milk, cheese and meat alternatives to find what works best for you. Try new recipes and dishes to keep things interesting.

5. **Get Support**: It may be helpful to get support from someone who also follows a vegan diet. Join a local vegan or vegetarian group.

Meal planning and preparation can help you stay on track with your vegan diet. Plan your meals, stock up on essentials, prepare meals, get creative, and get support. With time and effort, you can successfully transition to a plant-based lifestyle.

CHAPTER 6: BREAKFAST RECIPES

· Delicious and Healthy Breakfast Recipes

Try these delicious and healthy breakfast recipes.

1. **Overnight Oats**: Combine oats, chia seeds, blueberries, vanilla, almond milk, and maple syrup in an airtight container and store in the refrigerator overnight. In the morning, top with flaked almonds and half a banana and you're ready to go. If you want to eat something warm, heat it in the microwave for 1-2 minutes.

2. **Mango Overnight Oats**: These vegan overnight oats use a can of mango puree for an intense fruity flavor. It's different from normal breakfast.

3. **Spinach and Potato Cakes with Poached Eggs**: These Indian spiced spinach and potato cakes with melty poached eggs make a great meatless lunch or light dinner.

4. **Roasted Rhubarb and Oat Crumble with Greek Yogurt**: Start your day with sweet roasted rhubarb, orange pieces, creamy Greek yogurt and topped with a toasted oat crumble.

5. **Chilaquiles with Fresh Tomatillo Salsa**: Thomasina Miers' vegetarian chilaquiles are her interpretation of one of Mexico's most popular recipes. Top with a fried egg and enjoy for breakfast.

6. **Whiskey Jam**: James Strawbridge's classic jam will fill your kitchen with the scent of oranges and fill your cupboard with jars full of bittersweet goodness.

7. **Apple Cinnamon Porridge**: The best part about breakfast porridge is that you can add all your favorite ingredients. This recipe includes apples and cinnamon for a delicious and healthy start to your day.

8. **Banana Bread Smoothie**: This smoothie is the perfect way to start your day with nutritious ingredients like banana, Greek yogurt, and almond milk. Instructions:

a. Combine 1 ripe banana, 1/2 cup plain Greek yogurt, 1/2 cup unsweetened almond milk, 1/4 cup Old Fashioned rolled oats, 1 tablespoon honey, and 1/2 teaspoon of ground cinnamon in a blender.

b. Mix until a smooth and creamy mixture forms.

c. Pour into a glass and enjoy.

9. **Avocado Toast with Eggs**: This recipe is a classic breakfast staple that's easy to make and packed with healthy fats and protein.

Instructions:

a. Toast 1 slice of whole wheat bread.

b. Mash half an avocado and spread on toast.

c. Top with 1 fried egg and sprinkle with salt and pepper.

d. Serve and Enjoy

10. **Blueberry Chia Seed Pudding:** This recipe is a great way to get your daily dose of omega-3 fatty acids and antioxidants.

How to make:

a. In a bowl, combine 1/2 cup unsweetened almond milk, 1/2 cup plain Greek yogurt, 1/4 cup chia seeds, 1 tablespoon honey, and 1/2 teaspoon vanilla extract.

b. Let the mixture sit for 5 minutes and whisk again.

c. Cover and refrigerate for at least 2 hours or overnight.

d. Top with fresh blueberries and enjoy.

11. **Egg Muffins with Ham, Kale, and Cauliflower Rice**: These muffins are packed with vegetables and protein and are perfect for breakfast.

Directions:

a. Preheat oven to 375°F.

b. Coat a muffin tin with cooking spray.

c. In a large bowl, combine 8 eggs, 1/2 cup chopped kale, 1/2 cup cauliflower rice, 1/2 cup diced ham, 1/4 cup milk, 1/4 cup shredded cheddar cheese, and 1/2 teaspoon garlic powder. 1/2 teaspoon onion powder, 1/2 teaspoon salt, 1/4 teaspoon black pepper.

d. Pour the egg mixture into the prepared muffin tin.

e. Bake for 20-25 minutes or until muffins are set and golden brown.

f. Cool for 5 minutes before serving.

12. **Peanut Butter Banana Overnight Oats**: This recipe is perfect for busy mornings when you don't have time for breakfast.

How to make:

a. In a mason jar, combine 1/2 cup rolled oats, 1/2 cup unsweetened almond milk, 1/2 cup plain Greek yogurt, 1 tablespoon chia seeds, 1 tablespoon honey, 1/2 teaspoon vanilla extract, and 1/2 of a sliced banana.

b. Stir until everything is well mixed.

c. Cover and refrigerate overnight.

d. In the morning, add 1 tablespoon peanut butter and enjoy.

6. **Spinach and Feta Breakfast Wrap**: This recipe is a great way to get your daily dose of veggies and protein.

How to make:

a. In a small bowl, combine 2 eggs, 1/4 cup crumbled feta cheese, 1/4 cup chopped spinach, 1/4 teaspoon garlic powder, 1/4 teaspoon onion powder, 1/4 teaspoon salt, and 1/8 teaspoon Black pepper.

b. Heat a small nonstick frying pan over medium heat.

c. Pour the egg mixture into the saucepan and cook for 2 to 3 minutes or until the eggs are set.

d. Place the egg on top of the whole wheat wrap and roll it up.

e. Eat and enjoy

7. **Chocolate Chia Seed Pudding**: This recipe is a great way to satisfy your sweet tooth while still eating healthy.

How to make:

a. In a blender, combine 1 cup unsweetened almond milk, 1/4 cup chia seeds, 2 tablespoons cocoa powder, 2 tablespoons honey, and 1/2 teaspoon vanilla extract.

b. Mix until a smooth and creamy mixture forms.

c. Pour into a bowl and chill in the refrigerator for at least 2 hours or overnight.

d. Top with fresh berries and enjoy.

8. **Greek Yogurt Parfait**: This recipe is a quick and easy breakfast option rich in protein and fiber.

How to make:

a. In a bowl, layer 1 cup plain Greek yogurt, 1/2 cup fresh berries, and 1/4 cup granola.

b. Repeat layers until all ingredients are used.

c. Serve and Enjoy

9. **Sweet Potato Breakfast Hash**: This recipe is a hearty breakfast option perfect for meal prep.

How to make:

a. Preheat oven to 400°F.

b. Line a baking tray with baking paper.

c. In a large bowl, combine 2 cups diced sweet potatoes, 1 diced red bell pepper, 1 diced yellow onion, 2 minced garlic cloves, 2 tablespoons olive oil, 1 teaspoon smoked paprika, and 1/2 teaspoon salt, Add 1/4 teaspoon of black pepper and mix.

d. Spread the mixture evenly on the prepared baking sheet.

e. Bake for 20-25 minutes or until sweet potatoes are soft and golden brown.

f. Serve hot.

10. Green Smoothie Bowl: This recipe is a refreshing and nutritious breakfast option perfect for hot weather.

How to make:

a. Combine 1 frozen banana, 1/2 cup frozen mango, 1/2 cup frozen pineapple, 1/2 cup fresh spinach, 1/2 cup unsweetened almond milk, and 1 tablespoon honey in a blender.

b. Mix until a smooth and creamy mixture forms.

c. Pour the smoothie into a bowl and top with fresh fruit, granola, and chia seeds.

d. Enjoy

11. **Pumpkin Spice Overnight Oats**: This recipe is perfect for fall and winter mornings.

How to make:

a. In a mason jar, combine 1/2 cup rolled oats, 1/2 cup unsweetened almond milk, 1/4 cup canned pumpkin puree, 1 tablespoon maple syrup, 1/2 teaspoon pumpkin pie spice, and 1/2 cup teaspoons vanilla extract.

b. Stir until everything is well mixed.

c. Cover and refrigerate overnight.

d. Enjoy in the morning, topped with chopped pecans.

12. **Egg and Vegetable Breakfast Sandwich**: This recipe is a great way to get your daily dose of vegetables and protein.

How to make:

a. In a small nonstick skillet, sauté 1/4 cup sliced bell pepper and 1/4 cup sliced mushroom until soft.

b. In a separate bowl, combine 2 eggs, 1 tablespoon milk, and a pinch of salt and pepper.

c. Pour the egg mixture into the pot and cook until set.

d. Place eggs on whole wheat English muffins and top with sautéed vegetables.

e. Eat and enjoy

13. **Chocolate Peanut Butter Chia Seed Pudding**: This recipe is a great way to satisfy your sweet tooth while still eating healthy.

How to make:

a. In a blender, combine 1 cup unsweetened almond milk, 1/4 cup chia seeds, 2 tablespoons peanut butter, 2 tablespoons cocoa powder, 2 tablespoons honey, and 1/2 teaspoon vanilla extract.

b. Mix until a smooth and creamy mixture forms.

c. Pour into a bowl and chill in the refrigerator for at least 2 hours or overnight.

d. Top with fresh berries and enjoy.

14. **Healthy Breakfast Tacos**: This recipe is a fun and flavorful way to start your day.

How to make:

a. In a small nonstick skillet, fry 1/4 cup diced bell pepper and 1/4 cup chopped onion until soft.

b. In a separate bowl, combine 2 eggs, 1 tablespoon milk, and a pinch of salt and pepper.

c. Pour the egg mixture into the pot and cook until set.

d. Warm two small corn tortillas in the microwave or on the stove.

e. Place the egg on top of the tortilla, then top with 1/4 avocado, diced tomato, and a pinch of grated cheese.

f. Serve and Enjoy

15. **Healthy Breakfast Cookies**: This recipe is the perfect way to enjoy cookies for breakfast without feeling guilty.

How to make:

a. Preheat oven to 350°F.

b. Line a baking tray with baking paper.

c. Place 2 ripe bananas in a large bowl and mash with a fork.

d. Add 1 cup rolled oats, 1/2 cup unsweetened applesauce, 1/4 cup almond butter, 1/4 cup raisins, 1/4 cup chopped walnuts, 1 teaspoon cinnamon, and 1/2 teaspoon vanilla extract.

e. Stir until everything is well mixed.

f. Place spoonfuls of mixture on prepared baking sheet.

g. Bake for 15-20 minutes or until cookies are golden brown.

h. Let cool for 5 minutes before serving.

16. **Healthy Breakfast Sandwich**: This recipe is a great way to start your day with healthy protein and fiber.

How to make:

a. Toast a slice of whole wheat bread.

b. Spread 1 tablespoon of hummus on toast.

c. Top with 1 scrambled egg, 1 tomato slice, and a handful of baby spinach.

d. Sprinkle with salt and pepper.

e. Serve and enjoy.

17. **Overnight Oats with Peanut Butter and Jelly**: This recipe is a fun twist on the classic sandwich.

How to make:

a. In a mason jar, combine 1/2 cup rolled oats, 1/2 cup unsweetened almond milk, 1 tablespoon peanut butter, 1 tablespoon jelly, and 1/2 teaspoon vanilla extract.

b. Stir until everything is well mixed.

c. Cover and refrigerate overnight.

d. in the morning, topped with fresh berries and Enjoy

18. **Healthy Breakfast Burrito**: This recipe is a hearty and flavorful breakfast option that's perfect for meal prep.

How to make:

a. In a small nonstick skillet, fry 1/4 cup diced bell pepper and 1/4 cup chopped onion until soft.

b. In a separate bowl, combine 2 eggs, 1 tablespoon milk, and a pinch of salt and pepper.

c. Pour the egg mixture into the pot and cook until set.

d. Warm one small whole-wheat tortilla in the microwave or on the stove.

e. Place the egg on top of the tortilla, then top with a quarter of an avocado, diced tomatoes, and a pinch of grated cheese.

f. Roll and serve in tortillas

19. **Healthy Breakfast Bowl**: This recipe is a great way to get your daily dose of veggies and protein.

How to make:

a. In a bowl, combine 1/2 cup cooked quinoa, 1/2 cup sautéed kale, 1/4 cup black beans, 1/4 cup diced tomatoes, 1/4 avocado, and 1 fried egg.

b. Sprinkle with salt and pepper.

c. Enjoy

20. **Healthy Breakfast Cookies**: This recipe is the perfect way to enjoy cookies for breakfast without feeling guilty.

How to make:

a. Preheat oven to 350°F.

b. Line a baking tray with baking paper.

c. Place 2 ripe bananas in a large bowl and mash with a fork.

d. Add 1 cup rolled oats, 1/2 cup unsweetened applesauce, 1/4 cup almond butter, 1/4 cup raisins, 1/4 cup chopped walnuts, 1 teaspoon cinnamon, and 1/2 teaspoon vanilla extract.

e. Stir until everything is well mixed.

f. Place spoonfuls of mixture on prepared baking sheet.

g. Bake for 15-20 minutes or until cookies are golden brown.

h. Let cool for 5 minutes before serving.

21. **Healthy Breakfast Bars**: These bars are perfect for busy mornings when you don't have time to sit down and have breakfast.

How to make:

a. Preheat oven to 350°F.

b. Line a 20 x 20 cm baking dish with baking paper.

c. In a large bowl, combine 2 cups rolled oats, 1/2 cup chopped almonds, 1/2 cup dried cranberries, 1/4 cup honey, 1/4 cup melted coconut oil, 1 teaspoon vanilla extract, and salt 1/2 teaspoon .

d. Stir until everything is well mixed.

e. Press the mixture into the prepared baking dish.

f. Bake for 25-30 minutes or until bars are golden brown.

g. Let cool for 10 minutes before slicing and serving.

22. **Healthy Breakfast Smoothie**: This recipe is the perfect way to start your day with a nutritious and delicious smoothie.

How to make:

a. In a blender, combine 1 cup unsweetened almond milk, 1/2 cup frozen blueberries, 1/2 cup frozen strawberries, 1/2 frozen banana, 1/2 cup plain Greek yogurt, 1 tablespoon honey, and 1/2 teaspoon vanilla extract..

b. Mix until a smooth and creamy mixture forms.

c. Pour into a glass and enjoy.

23. **Healthy Breakfast Quesadillas**: This recipe is a fun and flavorful way to start your day.

How to make:

a. In a small nonstick skillet, fry 1/4 cup diced bell pepper and 1/4 cup chopped onion until soft.

b. In a separate bowl, combine 2 eggs, 1 tablespoon milk, and a pinch of salt and pepper.

c. Pour the egg mixture into the pot and cook until set.

d. Place the egg on a whole wheat tortilla and top with 1/4 cup of shredded cheddar cheese.

e. Cut the tortilla in half and fry in a pan until the cheese melts and the tortilla is golden brown.

f. Eat and enjoy

24. **Healthy Breakfast Muffins**: These muffins are a great way to start your day with a healthy dose of fiber and protein.

Directions:

a. Preheat oven to 375°F.

b. Line a muffin tin with paper liners.

c. In a large bowl, combine 2 cups almond flour, 1/2 cup oats, 1/4 cup honey, 1/4 cup melted coconut oil, 2 eggs, 1 teaspoon baking powder, 1/2 teaspoon baking soda, cinnamon 1/2 teaspoon and salt 1/4 teaspoon.

d. Stir in 1 cup fresh blueberries.

e. Divide batter evenly between prepared muffin cups.

f. Bake for 20 to 25 minutes or until muffins are golden brown and a toothpick inserted in the center comes out clean.

g. Let cool for 5 minutes before serving.

25. **Healthy Breakfast Pizza**: This recipe is a fun and creative way to start your day.

How to make:

a. Preheat oven to 425°F.

b. Spread 1 whole wheat pizza base onto a baking sheet.

c. Spread 1/4 cup tomato sauce over dough.

d. Top with 1/2 cup of shredded mozzarella cheese, 1/4 cup of diced bell pepper, 1/4 cup of chopped onion, and 2 scrambled eggs.

e. Bake for 12-15 minutes or until the crust is golden brown and the cheese is melted.

f. Slice and enjoy.

26. **Healthy Breakfast Tacos**: These tacos are a fun and flavorful way to start your day.

Directions:

a. In a small nonstick skillet, sauté 1/4 cup diced bell pepper and 1/4 cup chopped onion until soft.

b. In a separate bowl, combine 2 eggs, 1 tablespoon milk, and a pinch of salt and pepper.

c. Pour the egg mixture into the pot and cook until set.

d. Warm two small corn tortillas in the microwave or on the stove.

e. Place the egg on top of the tortilla, then top with 1/4 avocado, diced tomato, and a pinch of grated cheese.

f. Serve and Enjoy

27. **Healthy Breakfast Smoothie**: This smoothie is a perfect way to start his day with a nutritious and delicious drink.

How to make:

a. In a blender, combine 1 cup unsweetened almond milk, 1/2 cup frozen strawberries, 1/2 cup frozen blueberries, 1/2 frozen banana, 1/2 cup plain Greek yogurt, 1 tablespoon honey, and 1/2 teaspoon vanilla extract.

b. Mix until a smooth and creamy mixture forms.

c. Pour into a glass and enjoy.

28. **Healthy Breakfast Sandwich**: This sandwich is a great way to start your day with healthy protein and fiber.

How to make:

a. Toast a slice of whole wheat bread.

b. Spread 1 tablespoon of hummus on toast.

c. Top with 1 scrambled egg, 1 tomato slice, and a handful of baby spinach.

d. Sprinkle with salt and pepper.

e. Eat and Enjoy

29. **Healthy Breakfast Bowl**: This bowl is a great way to get your daily dose of veggies and protein.

How to make:

a. In a bowl, combine 1/2 cup cooked quinoa, 1/2 cup sautéed kale, 1/4 cup black beans, 1/4 cup diced tomatoes, 1/4 avocado, and 1 fried egg.

b. Sprinkle with salt and pepper.

c. Eat and Enjoy

30. **Healthy Breakfast Muffins**: These muffins are a great way to start your day with a healthy dose of fiber and protein.

Directions:

a. Preheat oven to 375°F.

b Line a muffin tin with paper liners.

c. In a large bowl, combine 2 cups almond flour, 1/2 cup oats, 1/4 cup honey, 1/4 cup melted coconut oil, 2 eggs, 1 teaspoon baking powder, 1/2 teaspoon baking soda, and 1/2 teaspoon baking soda and mix with 1/2 teaspoon cinnamon, 1/4 teaspoon salt.

d. Stir in 1 cup fresh blueberries.

e. Divide batter evenly between prepared muffin cups.

f. Bake for 20 to 25 minutes or until muffins are golden brown and a toothpick inserted in the center comes out clean.

g. Let cool for 5 minutes before serving.

31. **Healthy Breakfast Sandwich**: This sandwich is the perfect way to start your day with a healthy dose of protein and fiber.

How to make:

a. Toast a slice of whole wheat bread.

b. Spread 1 tablespoon of hummus on toast.

c. Top with 1 scrambled egg, 1 tomato slice, and a handful of baby spinach.

d. Sprinkle with salt and pepper.

e. Serve and Enjoy

32. **Healthy Breakfast Smoothie**: This smoothie is the perfect way to start your day with a nutritious and delicious drink.

How to make:

a. In a blender, combine 1 cup unsweetened almond milk, 1/2 cup frozen strawberries, 1/2 cup frozen blueberries, 1/2 frozen banana, 1/2 cup plain Greek yogurt, 1 tablespoon honey, and 1/2 teaspoon vanilla extract..

b. Mix until a smooth and creamy mixture forms.

c. Pour into a glass and enjoy.

33. **Healthy Breakfast Bowl**: This bowl is a great way to get your daily dose of vegetables and protein.

How to make:

a. In a bowl, combine 1/2 cup cooked quinoa, 1/2 cup sautéed kale, 1/4 cup black beans, 1/4 cup diced tomatoes, 1/4 avocado, and 1 fried egg.

b. Sprinkle with salt and pepper.

c. Eat and enjoy

34. **Healthy Breakfast Muffins**: These muffins are a great way to start your day with a healthy dose of fiber and protein.

Directions:

a. Preheat oven to 375°F.

b. Line a muffin tin with paper liners.

c. In a large bowl, combine 2 cups almond flour, 1/2 cup oats, 1/4 cup honey, 1/4 cup melted coconut oil, 2 eggs, 1 teaspoon baking powder, 1/2 teaspoon baking soda, and 1 cup baking soda.

Add /2 and mix. 1 teaspoon cinnamon, 1/4 teaspoon salt.

d. Stir in 1 cup fresh blueberries.

e. Divide batter evenly between prepared muffin cups.

f. Bake for 20 to 25 minutes or until muffins are golden brown and a toothpick inserted in the center comes out clean.

g. Let cool for 5 minutes before serving.

35. **Healthy Breakfast Pizza**: This pizza is a fun and creative way to start your day.

How to make:

a. Preheat oven to 425°F.

b. Spread 1 whole wheat pizza base onto a baking sheet.

c. Spread 1/4 cup tomato sauce over dough.

d. Top with 1/2 cup of shredded mozzarella cheese, 1/4 cup of diced bell pepper, 1/4 cup of chopped onion, and 2 scrambled eggs.

e. Bake for 12-15 minutes or until the crust is golden brown and the cheese is melted.

f. Slice and enjoy.

36. **Healthy Breakfast Smoothie**: This smoothie is a great way to start your day with a nutritious and delicious drink.

How to make:

a. In a blender, combine 1 cup unsweetened almond milk, 1/2 cup frozen strawberries, 1/2 cup frozen blueberries, 1/2 frozen banana, 1/2 cup plain Greek yogurt, 1 tablespoon honey, and 1/2 teaspoon vanilla extract.

b. Mix until a smooth and creamy mixture forms.

c. Pour into a glass and enjoy

37. **Healthy Breakfast Sandwich**: This sandwich is a great way to start your day with some healthy protein and fiber.

How to make:

a. Toast a slice of whole wheat bread.

b. Spread 1 tablespoon of hummus on toast.

c. Top with 1 scrambled egg, 1 tomato slice, and a handful of baby spinach.

d. Sprinkle with salt and pepper.

e. Eat and Enjoy

38. Healthy Breakfast Bowl: This bowl is a great way to get your daily dose of vegetables and protein.

How to make:

a. In a bowl, combine 1/2 cup cooked quinoa, 1/2 cup sautéed kale, 1/4 cup black beans, 1/4 cup diced tomatoes, 1/4 avocado, and 1 fried egg.

b. Sprinkle with salt and pepper.

c. Eat and Enjoy

39. **Healthy Breakfast Muffins**: These muffins are a great way to start your day with a healthy dose of fiber and protein.

Directions:

a. Preheat oven to 375°F.

b. Line a muffin tin with paper liners.

c. In a large bowl, combine 2 cups almond flour, 1/2 cup oats, 1/4 cup honey, 1/4 cup melted coconut oil, 2 eggs, 1 teaspoon baking powder, 1/2 teaspoon baking soda, and 1/2 teaspoon baking soda. 1/2 teaspoon cinnamon, 1/4 teaspoon salt.

d. Stir in 1 cup fresh blueberries.

e. Divide batter evenly between prepared muffin cups.

f. Bake for 20 to 25 minutes or until muffins are golden brown and a toothpick inserted in the center comes out clean.

g. Let cool for 5 minutes before serving.

40. **Healthy Breakfast Pizza**: This pizza is a fun and creative way to start your day.

How to make:

a. Preheat oven to 425°F.

b. Spread 1 whole wheat pizza base onto a baking sheet.

c. Spread 1/4 cup tomato sauce over dough.

d. Top with 1/2 cup of shredded mozzarella cheese, 1/4 cup of diced bell pepper, 1/4 cup of chopped onion, and 2 scrambled eggs.

e. Bake for 12-15 minutes or until the crust is golden brown and the cheese is melted.

f. Slice and enjoy.

41. **Healthy Breakfast Smoothie**: This smoothie is the perfect nutritious and delicious drink to start your day.

How to make:

a. In a blender, combine 1 cup unsweetened almond milk, 1/2

cup frozen strawberries, 1/2 cup frozen blueberries, 1/2 frozen banana, 1/2 cup plain Greek yogurt, 1 tablespoon honey, and 1/2 teaspoon vanilla extract.

b. Mix until a smooth and creamy mixture forms.

c. Pour into a glass and enjoy.

42. **Healthy Breakfast Sandwich**: This sandwich is a great way to start your day with healthy protein and fiber.

How to make:

a. Toast a slice of whole wheat bread.

b. Spread 1 tablespoon of hummus on toast.

c. Top with 1 scrambled egg, 1 tomato slice, and a handful of baby spinach.

d. Sprinkle with salt and pepper.

e. Serve and enjoy

43. **Healthy Breakfast Bowl**: This bowl is a great way to get your daily dose of vegetables and protein.

How to make:

a. In a bowl, combine 1/2 cup cooked quinoa, 1/2 cup sautéed kale, 1/4 cup black beans, 1/4 cup diced tomatoes, 1/4 avocado, and 1 fried egg.

b. Sprinkle with salt and pepper.

c. Eat and Enjoy

44. **Healthy Breakfast Muffins**: These muffins are a great way to start your day with a healthy dose of fiber and protein.

How to make:

a. Preheat oven to 375°F.

b. Line a muffin tin with paper liners.

c. In a large bowl, combine 2 cups almond flour, 1/2 cup oats, 1/4 cup honey, 1/4 cup melted coconut oil, 2 eggs, 1 teaspoon baking powder, 1/2 teaspoon baking soda, and 1 cup baking soda and mix 1/2 teaspoon cinnamon, 1/4 teaspoon salt.

d. Stir in 1 cup fresh blueberries.

e. Divide batter evenly between prepared muffin cups.

f. Bake for 20 to 25 minutes or until muffins are golden brown and a toothpick inserted in the center comes out clean.

g. Let cool for 5 minutes before serving.

45. **Healthy Breakfast Pizza**: This pizza is a fun and creative way to start your day.

How to make:

a. Preheat oven to 425°F.

b. Spread 1 whole wheat pizza base onto a baking sheet.

c. Spread 1/4 cup tomato sauce over the dough.

d. Top with 1/2 cup of shredded mozzarella cheese, 1/4 cup of diced bell pepper, 1/4 cup of chopped onion, and 2 scrambled eggs.

e. Bake for 12-15 minutes or until the crust is golden brown and the cheese is melted.

f. Slice and enjoy.

46. **Healthy Breakfast Burrito**: This burrito is a hearty and flavorful breakfast option perfect for meal prep.

How to make:

a. In a small nonstick skillet, fry 1/4 cup diced bell pepper and 1/4 cup chopped onion until soft.

b. In a separate bowl, combine 2 eggs, 1 tablespoon milk, and a pinch of salt and pepper.

c. Pour the egg mixture into the pot and cook until set.

d. Warm one small whole-wheat tortilla in the microwave or on the stove.

e. Place the egg on top of the tortilla and top with 1/4 cup of shredded cheddar cheese.

f. Cut the tortilla in half and fry in a pan until the cheese melts and the tortilla is golden brown.

g. Serve and Enjoy

47. **Healthy Breakfast Smoothie**: This smoothie is a perfect way to start his day with a nutritious and delicious drink.

How to make:

a. In a blender, combine 1 cup unsweetened almond milk, 1/2 cup frozen strawberries, 1/2 cup frozen blueberries, 1/2 frozen banana, 1/2 cup plain Greek yogurt, 1 tablespoon honey, and 1/2 teaspoon vanilla extract.

b. Mix until a smooth and creamy mixture forms.

c. Pour into a glass and enjoy

48. **Healthy Breakfast Smoothie**: This smoothie is the perfect nutritious and delicious drink to start your day.

How to make:

a. In a blender, combine 1 cup unsweetened almond milk, 1/2 cup frozen strawberries, 1/2 cup frozen blueberries, 1/2 frozen banana, 1/2 cup plain Greek yogurt, 1 tablespoon honey, and 1/2 teaspoon vanilla extract.

b. Mix until a smooth and creamy mixture forms.

c. Pour into a glass and enjoy.

49. **Healthy Breakfast Sandwich**: This sandwich is a great way to start your day with healthy protein and fiber.

How to make:

a. Toast a slice of whole wheat bread.

b. Spread 1 tablespoon of hummus on toast.

c. Top with 1 scrambled egg, 1 tomato slice, and a handful of baby spinach.

d. Sprinkle with salt and pepper.

e. Serve and Enjoy

50. **Healthy Breakfast Bowl**: This bowl is a great way to get your daily dose of vegetables and protein.

How to make:

a. In a bowl, combine 1/2 cup cooked quinoa, 1/2 cup sautéed kale, 1/4 cup black beans, 1/4 cup diced tomatoes, 1/4 avocado, and 1 fried egg.

b. Sprinkle with salt and pepper.

c. Eat and Enjoy

51. **Healthy Breakfast Muffins**: These muffins are a great way to start your day with a healthy dose of fiber and protein.

Directions:

a. Preheat oven to 375°F.

b. Line a muffin tin with paper liners.

c. In a large bowl, combine 2 cups almond flour, 1/2 cup oats, 1/4 cup honey, 1/4 cup melted coconut oil, 2 eggs, 1 teaspoon baking powder, 1/2 teaspoon baking soda, and 1 cup baking soda.

Add /2 and mix.

1 teaspoon cinnamon, 1/4 teaspoon salt.

d. Stir in 1 cup fresh blueberries.

e. Divide batter evenly between prepared muffin cups.

f. Bake for 20 to 25 minutes or until muffins are golden brown and a toothpick inserted in the center comes out clean.

g. Let cool for 5 minutes before serving.

52. **Healthy Breakfast Pizza**: This pizza is a fun and creative way to start your day.

How to make:

a. Preheat oven to 425°F.

b. Spread 1 whole wheat pizza base onto a baking sheet.

c. Spread 1/4 cup tomato sauce over dough.

d. Top with 1/2 cup of shredded mozzarella cheese, 1/4 cup of diced bell pepper, 1/4 cup of chopped onion, and 2 scrambled eggs.

e. Bake for 12-15 minutes or until the crust is golden brown and the cheese is melted.

f. Slice and enjoy.

53. **Healthy Breakfast Burrito**: This burrito is a hearty and flavorful breakfast option perfect for meal prep.

How to make:

a. In a small nonstick skillet, fry 1/4 cup diced bell pepper and 1/4 cup chopped onion until soft.

b. In a separate bowl, combine 2 eggs, 1 tablespoon milk, and a pinch of salt and pepper.

c. Pour the egg mixture into the pot and cook until set.

d. Warm one small whole-wheat tortilla in the microwave or on the stove.

e. Place the egg on top of the tortilla and top with 1/4 cup of shredded cheddar cheese.

f. Cut the tortillas in half and cook in a pan until the cheese melts and the tortillas are golden brown.

g. Serve and Enjoy

54. **Healthy Breakfast Smoothie**: This smoothie is the perfect way to start your day with a nutritious and delicious drink.

How to make:

a. In a blender, combine 1 cup unsweetened almond milk, 1/2 cup frozen strawberries, 1/2 cup frozen blueberries, 1/2 frozen banana, 1/2 cup plain Greek yogurt, 1 tablespoon honey, and 1/2 teaspoon vanilla extract.

b. Mix until a smooth and creamy mixture forms.

c. Pour into a glass and enjoy.

55. **Healthy Breakfast Smoothie**: This smoothie is the perfect nutritious and delicious drink to start your day.

How to make:

a. In a blender, combine 1 cup unsweetened almond milk, 1/2 cup frozen strawberries, 1/2 cup frozen blueberries, 1/2 frozen banana, 1/2 cup plain Greek yogurt, 1 tablespoon honey, and 1/2 teaspoon vanilla extract.

b. Mix until a smooth and creamy mixture forms.

c. Pour into a glass and enjoy

56. **Healthy Breakfast Sandwich**: This sandwich is a great way to start your day with healthy protein and fiber.

How to make:

a. Toast a slice of whole wheat bread.

b. Spread 1 tablespoon of hummus on toast.

c. Top with 1 scrambled egg, 1 tomato slice, and a handful of baby spinach.

d. Sprinkle with salt and pepper.

e. Eat and Enjoy

57. **Healthy Breakfast Bowl**: This bowl is a great way to get your daily dose of veggies and protein.

How to make:

a. In a bowl, combine 1/2 cup cooked quinoa, 1/2 cup sautéed kale, 1/4 cup black beans, 1/4 cup diced tomatoes, 1/4 avocado, and 1 fried egg.

b. Sprinkle with salt and pepper.

c. Serve and enjoy

58. **Healthy Breakfast Muffins**: These muffins are a great way to start your day with a healthy amount of fiber and protein.

Directions:

a. Preheat oven to 375°F.

b. Line a muffin tin with paper liners.

c. In a large bowl, combine 2 cups almond flour, 1/2 cup oats, 1/4 cup honey, 1/4 cup melted coconut oil, 2 eggs, 1 teaspoon baking powder, 1/2 teaspoon baking soda, and 1 cup baking soda.

Add /2 and mix.

1 teaspoon cinnamon, 1/4 teaspoon salt.

d. Stir in 1 cup fresh blueberries.

e. Divide batter evenly between prepared muffin cups.

f. Bake for 20 to 25 minutes or until muffins are golden brown and a toothpick inserted in the center comes out clean.

g. Let cool for 5 minutes before serving.

59. **Healthy Breakfast Pizza**: This pizza is a fun and creative way to start your day.

How to make:

a. Preheat oven to 425°F.

b. Spread 1 whole wheat pizza base onto a baking sheet.

c. Spread 1/4 cup tomato sauce over dough.

d. Top with 1/2 cup of shredded mozzarella cheese, 1/4 cup of diced bell pepper, 1/4 cup of chopped onion, and 2 scrambled eggs.

e. Bake for 12-15 minutes or until the crust is golden brown and the cheese is melted.

f. Slice and enjoy.

60. **Healthy Breakfast Burrito**: This burrito is a hearty and flavorful breakfast option perfect for meal prep.

How to make:

a. In a small nonstick skillet, fry 1/4 cup diced bell pepper and 1/4 cup chopped onion until soft.

b. In a separate bowl, combine 2 eggs, 1 tablespoon milk, and a pinch of salt and pepper.

c. Pour the egg mixture into the pot and cook until set.

d. Warm one small whole-wheat tortilla in the microwave or on the stove.

e. Place the egg on top of the tortilla and top with 1/4 cup of shredded cheddar cheese.

f. Cut the tortillas in half and cook in a pan until the cheese melts and the tortillas are golden brown.

g. Serve and enjoy

CHAPTER 7: LUNCH RECIPES

· Delicious and Healthy Lunch Recipes

1. **Vegan Caesar Salad**: This salad is a great way to get your daily dose of vegetables.

For the dressing, combine 1/4 cup tahini, 1/4 cup lemon juice, 2 garlic cloves, 1 tablespoon Dijon mustard, 1 tablespoon nutritional yeast, 1/4 teaspoon salt, and 1/4 teaspoon black pepper in a blender. Stir everything until smooth. Mix dressing with chopped romaine lettuce, croutons, and vegan Parmesan. Enjoy!

2. **Vegan BLT Sandwich**: This sandwich is a classic lunchtime favorite. For sandwiches, toast two slices of bread. Spread vegan mayonnaise on a slice of bread and top with lettuce, tomato, and eggplant bacon. Top with another slice of bread and enjoy.

3. **Vegan Lentil Soup**: This soup is hearty and filling. To make the soup, heat 1 tablespoon of the olive oil in a large pot over medium heat. Add 1 chopped onion, 2 chopped carrots, and 2 chopped celery sticks.

Cook until the vegetables are soft. Add 2 minced garlic cloves and cook for 1 minute. Add 1 cup dried lentils, 4 cups vegetable broth, 1 can diced tomatoes, 1 teaspoon dried thyme, 1 teaspoon dried oregano, 1/2 teaspoon salt, and 1/4 teaspoon black pepper. Once it boils, reduce the heat and simmer for about 30 minutes. Enjoy!

4. **Vegan Chickpea Salad**: This salad is high in protein. To make the salad, use 1 can of chickpeas (drained and washed), 1 diced red bell pepper, 1 diced yellow bell pepper, 1 diced cucumber, and 1/4 chopped red onion, 1/4 cup chopped fresh parsley in a large bowl. In a separate bowl, combine 1/4 cup olive oil, 2 tablespoons lemon juice, 1 minced garlic clove, 1/2 teaspoon salt, and 1/4

teaspoon black pepper. Pour dressing over salad and mix. enjoy!

5. **Vegan Tofu Bread**: This bread is quick and easy to prepare.

To make the stir-fry, heat 1 tablespoon of vegetable oil in a large skillet over high heat. Add 1 minced onion, 2 minced garlic cloves and 1 minced red chili pepper. Cook until the vegetables are soft. Add 1 cubed tofu and fry until the tofu turns golden brown. Add 1/4 cup soy sauce, 1 tablespoon maple syrup, and 1 tablespoon cornstarch. Simmer until the sauce thickens. Enjoy with rice!

6. **Vegan Tuna Salad**: This salad is a great way to get your daily dose of protein. To prepare the salad: 1 can chickpeas (drained and washed), 1/4 cup vegan mayonnaise, 1 tablespoon Dijon mustard, 1 tablespoon nutritional yeast, 1/4 teaspoon salt, 1/4 teaspoon black pepper Place in a large bowl. Mash the chickpeas with a fork until they crumble. Add chopped celery, chopped red onion, and chopped cucumber. Mix well and enjoy!

7. **Vegan Caesar Wrap**: This wrap is the perfect way to enjoy a classic salad in a portable form. For wraps, spread vegan Caesar dressing on a large tortilla. Top with shredded romaine lettuce, vegan Parmesan cheese, and croutons. Wrap it in a tortilla and enjoy!

8. **Vegan BLT Salad**: This salad is a deconstructed version of the classic sandwich. For the salad, cut lettuce and tomatoes. Add crumbled eggplant bacon and vegan mayonnaise. Mix well and enjoy!

9. **Vegan Lentil Salad**: This salad is packed with protein and fiber. For a salad, cook 1 cup of lentils according to package directions. Drain and wash the lentils. Add diced cucumber, diced red onion, diced red bell pepper, and chopped fresh parsley. In a separate bowl, combine 1/4 cup olive oil, 2 tablespoons lemon juice, 1 minced garlic clove, 1/2 teaspoon salt, and 1/4 teaspoon black pepper. Pour dressing over salad and mix. enjoy!

10. **Vegan Chickpea Curry**: A hearty curry. To make the curry, heat

1 tablespoon of vegetable oil in a large pot over medium heat. Add 1 minced onion and 2 minced garlic cloves. Cook until onions are soft. Add 2 tablespoons of curry powder and simmer for 1 minute. Add 2 cans of chickpeas (drained and ashed), 1 can of diced tomatoes, and 1 can of coconut milk. Once it boils, reduce the heat and simmer or 15 minutes. Enjoy with rice!

11. **Vegan Greek Salad**: The perfect salad to enjoy the flavors of Greece. For the salad, cut lettuce, omato, cucumber, and red onion. Add sliced kalamata olives and crumbled vegan feta cheese. Drizzle with olive oil and red wine vinegar. Mix well and enjoy!

12. **Vegan Falafel Wrap**: This wrap is the perfect way to enjoy the flavors of the Middle East. For the wrap, spread hummus on a large tortilla. Top with falafel balls, chopped lettuce, diced tomatoes, and diced cucumber. Wrap it in a tortilla and enjoy!

13. **Vegan Black Bean Soup**: This soup is hearty and filling. To make the soup, heat 1 tablespoon of the olive oil in a large pot over medium heat. Add 1 chopped onion, 2 chopped carrots, and 2 chopped celery sticks. Cook until the vegetables are soft. Add 2 minced garlic cloves and cook for 1 minute. Add 2 cans of black beans (drained and washed), 4 cups of vegetable broth, 1 can of diced tomatoes, 1 teaspoon of ground cumin, 1/2 teaspoon of salt, and 1/4 teaspoon of black pepper. Once it boils, reduce the heat and simmer for about 30 minutes. enjoy!

14. **Vegan Capri Salad**: The perfect salad to enjoy the flavors of Italy. For the salad, slice tomatoes and vegan mozzarella. Arrange the slices on a plate. Serve with olive oil and balsamic vinegar. Sprinkle with chopped fresh basil. enjoy!

15. **Vegan Sweet Potato Chili**: This chili is hearty and filling. To prepare chili peppers, heat 1 tablespoon vegetable oil in a large pot over medium-high heat. Add 1 minced onion and 2 minced garlic cloves. Cook until onions are soft. Add 2 chopped sweet potatoes, 1 can diced tomatoes, 1 can black beans (drained and washed), 1 tablespoon chili powder, 1 teaspoon ground cumin, 1/2 teaspoon

salt, and 1/4 teaspoon black pepper. Add enough water to cover the vegetables. Once it boils, reduce the heat and simmer for about 30 minutes. enjoy!

8. **Vegan BLT Salad**: This salad is a deconstructed version of the classic sandwich. For the salad, cut lettuce and tomatoes. Add crumbled eggplant bacon and vegan mayonnaise. Mix well and enjoy!

9.   **Vegan Lentil Salad**: This salad is packed with protein and fiber. For a salad, cook 1 cup of lentils according to package directions. Drain and wash the lentils. Add diced cucumber, diced red onion, diced red bell pepper, and chopped fresh parsley. In a separate bowl, combine 1/4 cup olive oil, 2 tablespoons lemon juice, 1 minced garlic clove, 1/2 teaspoon salt, and 1/4 teaspoon black pepper. Pour dressing over salad and mix. enjoy!

10. **Vegan Chickpea Curry**: A hearty curry. To make the curry, heat 1 tablespoon of vegetable oil in a large pot over medium heat. Include 1 minced onion and 2 minced garlic cloves. Cook until onions are soft. Add 2 tablespoons of curry powder and simmer for 1 minute. Add 2 cans of chickpeas (drained and washed), 1 can of diced tomatoes, and 1 can of coconut milk. Once it boils, reduce the heat and simmer for 15 minutes. Enjoy with rice!

11. **Vegan Greek Salad**: The perfect salad to enjoy the flavors of Greece. For the salad, cut lettuce, tomato, cucumber, and red onion. Add sliced kalamata olives and crumbled vegan feta cheese. Coat with olive oil and red wine vinegar. Mix well and enjoy!

12. **Vegan Falafel Wrap**: This wrap is the perfect way to enjoy the flavors of the Middle East. For the wrap, spread hummus on a large tortilla. Top with falafel balls, chopped lettuce, diced tomatoes, and diced cucumber. Wrap it in a tortilla and enjoy!

13. **Vegan Black Bean Soup**: This soup is hearty and filling. To make the soup, heat 1 tablespoon of the olive oil in a large pot over medium heat. Add 1 chopped onion, 2 chopped carrots, and 2 chopped celery sticks. Cook until the vegetables are soft. Add 2 minced garlic cloves and cook for 1 minute. Add 2 cans of black beans (drained and washed), 4 cups of vegetable broth, 1 can of diced tomatoes, 1 teaspoon of ground cumin, 1/2 teaspoon of salt, and 1/4 teaspoon of black pepper. Once it boils, reduce the heat and simmer for about 30 minutes. enjoy!

14. **Vegan Capri Salad**: The perfect salad to enjoy the flavors of Italy. For the salad, slice tomatoes and vegan mozzarella. Arrange the slices on a plate. Serve with olive oil and balsamic vinegar. Sprinkle with chopped fresh basil. enjoy!

15. **Vegan Sweet Potato Chili**: This chili is hearty and filling. To prepare chili peppers, heat 1 tablespoon vegetable oil in a large pot over medium-high heat. Include 1 minced onion and 2 minced garlic cloves. Cook until onions are soft. Add 2 chopped sweet potatoes, 1 can diced tomatoes, 1 can black beans (drained and washed), 1 tablespoon chili powder, 1 teaspoon ground cumin, 1/2 teaspoon salt, and 1/4 teaspoon black pepper. Add enough water to cover the vegetables. Once it boils, reduce the heat and simmer for about 30 minutes. enjoy!

16. **Vegan Chickpea Tacos**: These tacos are a great way to enjoy a plant-based meal. To prepare tacos, heat 1 tablespoon vegetable oil in a large skillet over medium-high heat. Add 1 minced onion, 2 minced garlic cloves and 1 minced red chili pepper. Cook until the vegetables are soft. Add 1 can of chickpeas (drained and washed), 1 tablespoon chili powder, 1 teaspoon cumin powder, 1/2 teaspoon salt, and 1/4 teaspoon black pepper. Boil until the chickpeas are cooked through. Serve in taco shells.

17. **Vegan Greek Pasta Salad**: This salad is a great way to enjoy the flavors of Greece. To prepare the salad, cook 8 ounces of pasta according to package directions. Drain and wash the noodles. Add

chopped cucumber, chopped red onion, chopped kalamata olives, and crumbled vegan feta cheese. In a separate bowl, combine 1/4 cup olive oil, 2 tablespoons red wine vinegar, 1 minced garlic clove, 1/2 teaspoon dried oregano, 1/4 teaspoon salt, and 1/4 teaspoon black pepper. Pour dressing over salad and mix. enjoy!

18. **Vegan Lentil Sloppy Joes**: These Sloppy Joes are the perfect way to enjoy a classic sandwich. To make slew joes, heat 1 tablespoon of olive oil in a large skillet over medium-high heat. Add 1 chopped onion and 2 minced garlic cloves. Cook until onions are soft. Add 1 can of lentils (drained and washed), 1 can of tomato sauce, 1 tablespoon of maple syrup, 1 tablespoon of Dijon mustard, 1 tablespoon of apple cider vinegar, 1 teaspoon of chili powder, and 1/2 teaspoon of salt. 1/4 teaspoon black pepper. Cook until heated through. Wrap it in a bread roll and enjoy!

19. **Vegan Chickpea Salad Sandwich**: This sandwich is a great way to enjoy a protein-packed lunch. To make the sandwich, mash 1 can of chickpeas (drained and washed) with a fork. Add 1/4 cup vegan mayonnaise, 1 tablespoon Dijon mustard, 1 tablespoon nutritional yeast, 1/4 teaspoon salt, and 1/4 teaspoon black pepper. Mix well. Spread the chickpea salad on bread and top with lettuce, tomato, and avocado. Top with another slice of bread and enjoy.

20. **Vegan Quinoa Salad**: This salad is packed with protein and fiber. For the salad, cook 1 cup of quinoa according to package directions. Drain and wash the quinoa. Add diced cucumber, diced red onion, diced red bell pepper, and chopped fresh parsley. In a separate bowl, combine 1/4 cup olive oil, 2 tablespoons lemon juice, 1 minced garlic clove, 1/2 teaspoon salt, and 1/4 teaspoon black pepper. Pour dressing over salad and mix. enjoy!

21. **Vegan Buffalo Cauliflower Wraps**: These wraps are a great way to enjoy the flavor of buffalo sauce.

To prepare the wraps, preheat the oven to 200°C. Cut 1 cauliflower into florets. In a large bowl, combine 1/4 cup hot sauce, 2 tablespoons melted vegan butter, 1 tablespoon apple cider vinegar, 1/2 teaspoon garlic powder, and 1/4 teaspoon salt. Add the cauliflower florets and mix. Spread the cauliflower on a baking sheet and bake for 20 minutes. To assemble wraps, spread vegan ranch dressing onto a large tortilla. Top with roasted cauliflower, chopped lettuce, and diced tomatoes. Wrap it in a tortilla and enjoy!

22. **Vegan Chickpea Noodle Soup**: This soup is hearty and filling. To make the soup, heat 1 tablespoon of the olive oil in a large pot over medium heat. Add 1 chopped onion, 2 chopped carrots, and 2 chopped celery sticks. Cook until the vegetables are soft. Add 2 minced garlic cloves and cook for 1 minute. Add 1 can of chickpeas (drained and washed), 4 cups of vegetable broth, 1 cup of cooked pasta, 1 teaspoon of dried thyme, 1/2 teaspoon of salt, and 1/4 teaspoon of black pepper. Once it boils, reduce the heat and simmer for about 30 minutes. enjoy!

23. **Vegan Falafel Salad**: This salad is a great way to enjoy the flavors of the Middle East. To make the salad, combine chopped lettuce, diced tomatoes, diced cucumber, and red onion slices in a large bowl. Add falafel balls and drizzle with tahini dressing. enjoy!

24. **Vegan Chickpea Tuna Melt**: This sandwich is a great way to enjoy a classic tuna melt. To make the sandwich, mash 1 can of chickpeas (drained and washed) with a fork. Add 1/4 cup vegan mayonnaise, 1 tablespoon Dijon mustard, 1 tablespoon nutritional yeast, 1/4 teaspoon salt, and 1/4 teaspoon black pepper. Mix well. Spread the chickpea salad on bread and top with vegan cheese. Bake until the cheese is melted. enjoy!

25. **Vegan Greek Pasta**: This pasta dish is the perfect way to enjoy the flavors of Greece. To prepare pasta, cook 8 ounces of pasta according to package directions. Drain and wash the noodles. Add chopped cucumber, chopped red onion, chopped kalamata olives, and crumbled vegan feta cheese. In a separate bowl, combine 1/4

cup olive oil, 2 tablespoons red wine vinegar, 1 minced garlic clove, 1/2 teaspoon dried oregano, 1/4 teaspoon salt, and 1/4 teaspoon black pepper. Pour dressing over pasta and mix. enjoy!

26. **Vegan Chickpea Salad**: This salad is rich in protein. To make the salad, use 1 can of chickpeas (drained and washed), 1 diced red bell pepper, 1 diced yellow bell pepper, 1 diced cucumber, and 1/4 chopped red onion. Cup, 1/4 cup chopped fresh parsley in a large bowl. In a separate bowl, combine 1/4 cup olive oil, 2 tablespoons lemon juice, 1 minced garlic clove, 1/2 teaspoon salt, and 1/4 teaspoon black pepper. Pour dressing over salad and mix. enjoy!

27. **Vegan Lentil Soup**: This soup is hearty and filling. To make the soup, heat 1 tablespoon of the olive oil in a large pot over medium heat. Add 1 chopped onion, 2 chopped carrots, and 2 chopped celery sticks. Cook until the vegetables are soft. Add 2 minced garlic cloves and cook for 1 minute. Add 1 cup dried lentils, 4 cups vegetable broth, 1 can diced tomatoes, 1 teaspoon dried thyme, 1 teaspoon dried oregano, 1/2 teaspoon salt, and 1/4 teaspoon black pepper. Once it boils, reduce the heat and simmer for about 30 minutes. enjoy!

28. **Vegan Chickpea Salad Sandwich**: This sandwich is a great way to enjoy a protein-packed lunch. To make the sandwich, mash 1 can of chickpeas (drained and washed) with a fork. Add 1/4 cup vegan mayonnaise, 1 tablespoon Dijon mustard, 1 tablespoon nutritional yeast, 1/4 teaspoon salt, and 1/4 teaspoon black pepper. Mix well. Spread the chickpea salad on bread and top with lettuce, tomato, and avocado. Top with another slice of bread and enjoy.

29. **Vegan Quinoa Salad**: This salad is packed with protein and fiber. For the salad, cook 1 cup of quinoa according to package directions. Drain and wash the quinoa. Add diced cucumber, diced red onion, diced red bell pepper, and chopped fresh parsley. In a separate bowl, combine 1/4 cup olive oil, 2 tablespoons lemon

juice, 1 minced garlic clove, 1/2 teaspoon salt, and 1/4 teaspoon black pepper. Pour dressing over salad and mix. enjoy!

30. **Vegan Buffalo Cauliflower Tacos**: These tacos are a great way to enjoy the flavor of buffalo sauce. To prepare tacos, preheat oven to 425°F. Cut 1 cauliflower into florets. In a large bowl, combine 1/4 cup hot sauce, 2 tablespoons melted vegan butter, 1 tablespoon apple cider vinegar, 1/2 teaspoon garlic powder, and 1/4 teaspoon salt. Add the cauliflower florets and mix. Spread the cauliflower on a baking sheet and bake for 20 minutes. To assemble tacos, brush tortillas with vegan ranch dressing. Top with roasted cauliflower, chopped lettuce, and diced tomatoes. enjoy!

31. **Vegan Chickpea Lettuce Wraps**: These wraps are a great way to enjoy a protein-packed lunch. For the wrap, mash 1 can of chickpeas (drained and washed) with a fork. Add 1/4 cup vegan mayonnaise, 1 tablespoon Dijon mustard, 1 tablespoon nutritional yeast, 1/4 teaspoon salt, and 1/4 teaspoon black pepper. Mix well. Spread the chickpea salad onto tortillas and top with lettuce, tomato, and avocado. Wrap it in a tortilla and enjoy!

32. **Vegan Greek Lettuce Wrap**: This wrap is the perfect way to enjoy the flavors of Greece. For wraps, spread hummus on tortillas. Top with shredded lettuce, diced tomatoes, sliced kalamata olives, and crumbled vegan feta cheese. Wrap it in a tortilla and enjoy!

27. **Vegan Lentil Soup**: This soup is hearty and filling. To make the soup, heat 1 tablespoon of the olive oil in a large pot over medium heat. Add 1 chopped onion, 2 chopped carrots, and 2 chopped celery sticks. Cook until the vegetables are soft. Add 2 minced garlic cloves and cook for 1 minute. Add 1 cup dried lentils, 4 cups vegetable broth, 1 can diced tomatoes, 1 teaspoon dried thyme, 1 teaspoon dried oregano, 1/2 teaspoon salt, and 1/4 teaspoon black pepper. Once it boils, reduce the heat and simmer for about 30 minutes. enjoy!

28. **Vegan Chickpea Salad Sandwich**: This sandwich is a great way to enjoy a protein-packed lunch. To make the sandwich, mash 1 can of chickpeas (drained and washed) with a fork. Add 1/4 cup vegan mayonnaise, 1 tablespoon Dijon mustard, 1 tablespoon nutritional yeast, 1/4 teaspoon salt, and 1/4 teaspoon black pepper. Mix well. Spread the chickpea salad on bread and top with lettuce, tomato, and avocado. Top with another slice of bread and enjoy.

29. **Vegan Quinoa Salad**: This salad is packed with protein and fiber. For the salad, cook 1 cup of quinoa according to package directions. Drain and wash the quinoa. Add diced cucumber, diced red onion, diced red bell pepper, and chopped fresh parsley. In a separate bowl, combine 1/4 cup olive oil, 2 tablespoons lemon juice, 1 minced garlic clove, 1/2 teaspoon salt, and 1/4 teaspoon black pepper. Pour dressing over salad and mix. enjoy!

30. **Vegan Buffalo Cauliflower Tacos**: These tacos are a great way to enjoy the flavor of buffalo sauce. To prepare tacos, preheat oven to 425°F. Cut 1 cauliflower into florets. In a large bowl, combine 1/4 cup hot sauce, 2 tablespoons melted vegan butter, 1 tablespoon apple cider vinegar, 1/2 teaspoon garlic powder, and 1/4 teaspoon salt. Add the cauliflower florets and mix. Spread the cauliflower on a baking sheet and bake for 20 minutes. To assemble tacos, brush tortillas with vegan ranch dressing. Top with roasted cauliflower, chopped lettuce, and diced tomatoes. enjoy!

31. **Vegan Chickpea Lettuce Wraps**: These wraps are a great way to enjoy a protein-packed lunch. For the wrap, mash 1 can of chickpeas (drained and washed) with a fork. Add 1/4 cup vegan mayonnaise, 1 tablespoon Dijon mustard, 1 tablespoon nutritional yeast, 1/4 teaspoon salt, and 1/4 teaspoon black pepper. Mix well. Spread the chickpea salad onto tortillas and top with lettuce, tomato, and avocado. Wrap it in a tortilla and enjoy!

32. **Vegan Greek Lettuce Wrap**: This wrap is the perfect way

to enjoy the flavors of Greece. For wraps, spread hummus on tortillas. Top with shredded lettuce, diced tomatoes, sliced kalamata olives, and crumbled vegan feta cheese. Wrap it in a tortilla and enjoy!

39. **Vegan Greek Pasta**: This pasta dish is the perfect way to enjoy the flavors of Greece. To prepare pasta, cook 8 ounces of pasta according to package directions. Drain and wash the noodles. Add chopped cucumber, chopped red onion, chopped kalamata olives, and crumbled vegan feta cheese. In a separate bowl, combine 1/4 cup olive oil, 2 tablespoons red wine vinegar, 1 minced garlic clove, 1/2 teaspoon dried oregano, 1/4 teaspoon salt, and 1/4 teaspoon black pepper. Pour dressing over pasta and mix. enjoy!

40. **Vegan Chickpea Salad**: This salad is rich in protein. To make the salad, use 1 can of chickpeas (drained and washed), 1 diced red bell pepper, 1 diced yellow bell pepper, 1 diced cucumber, and 1/4 chopped red onion. Cup, 1/4 cup chopped fresh parsley in a large bowl. In a separate bowl, combine 1/4 cup olive oil, 2 tablespoons lemon juice, 1 minced garlic clove, 1/2 teaspoon salt, and 1/4 teaspoon black pepper. Pour dressing over salad and mix. enjoy!

41. **Vegan Lentil Soup**: This soup is hearty and filling. To make the soup, heat 1 tablespoon of the olive oil in a large pot over medium heat. Add 1 chopped onion, 2 chopped carrots, and 2 chopped celery sticks. Cook until the vegetables are soft. Add 2 minced garlic cloves and cook for 1 minute. Add 1 cup dried lentils, 4 cups vegetable broth, 1 can diced tomatoes, 1 teaspoon dried thyme, 1 teaspoon dried oregano, 1/2 teaspoon salt, and 1/4 teaspoon black pepper. Once it boils, reduce the heat and simmer for about 30 minutes. enjoy!

42. **Vegan Chickpea Salad Sandwich**: This sandwich is a great way to enjoy a protein-packed lunch. To make the sandwich, mash 1 can of chickpeas (drained and washed) with a fork. Add 1/4 cup vegan mayonnaise, 1 tablespoon Dijon mustard, 1 tablespoon nutritional yeast, 1/4 teaspoon salt, and 1/4 teaspoon black

pepper. Mix well. Spread the chickpea salad on bread and top with lettuce, tomato, and avocado. Top with another slice of bread and enjoy.

43. **Vegan Quinoa Salad**: This salad is packed with protein and fiber. For the salad, cook 1 cup of quinoa according to package directions. Drain and wash the quinoa. Add diced cucumber, diced red onion, diced red bell pepper, and chopped fresh parsley. In a separate bowl, combine 1/4 cup olive oil, 2 tablespoons lemon juice, 1 minced garlic clove, 1/2 teaspoon salt, and 1/4 teaspoon black pepper. Pour dressing over salad and mix. enjoy!

44. **Vegan Buffalo Cauliflower Wraps**: These wraps are a great way to enjoy the flavor of buffalo sauce. To prepare the wraps, preheat the oven to 200°C. Cut 1 cauliflower into florets. In a large bowl, combine 1/4 cup hot sauce, 2 tablespoons melted vegan butter, 1 tablespoon apple cider vinegar, 1/2 teaspoon garlic powder, and 1/4 teaspoon salt. Add the cauliflower florets and mix. Spread the cauliflower on a baking sheet and bake for 20 minutes. To assemble wraps, spread vegan ranch dressing onto a large tortilla. Top with roasted cauliflower, chopped lettuce, and diced tomatoes. Wrap it in a tortilla and enjoy!

45. **Vegan Chickpea Noodle Soup**: This soup is hearty and filling. To make the soup, heat 1 tablespoon of the olive oil in a large pot over medium heat. Add 1 chopped onion, 2 chopped carrots, and 2 chopped celery sticks. Cook until the vegetables are soft. Add 2 minced garlic cloves and cook for 1 minute. Add 1 can of chickpeas (drained and washed), 4 cups of vegetable broth, 1 cup of cooked pasta, 1 teaspoon of dried thyme, 1/2 teaspoon of salt, and 1/4 teaspoon of black pepper. Once it boils, reduce the heat and simmer for about 30 minutes. enjoy!

46. **Vegan Falafel Salad**: This salad is a great way to enjoy the flavors of the Middle East. To make the salad, combine chopped lettuce, diced tomatoes, diced cucumber, and red onion slices in

a large bowl. Add falafel balls and drizzle with tahini dressing. enjoy!

47. **Vegan Chickpea Tuna Melt**: This sandwich is a great way to enjoy a classic tuna melt. To make the sandwich, mash 1 can of chickpeas (drained and washed) with a fork. Add 1/4 cup vegan mayonnaise, 1 tablespoon Dijon mustard, 1 tablespoon nutritional yeast, 1/4 teaspoon salt, and 1/4 teaspoon black pepper. Mix well. Spread the chickpea salad on bread and top with vegan cheese. Bake until the cheese is melted. enjoy!

48. **Vegan Greek Pasta**: This pasta dish is the perfect way to enjoy the flavors of Greece. To prepare pasta, cook 8 ounces of pasta according to package directions. Drain and wash the noodles. Add chopped cucumber, chopped red onion, chopped kalamata olives, and crumbled vegan feta cheese. In a separate bowl, combine 1/4 cup olive oil, 2 tablespoons red wine vinegar, 1 minced garlic clove, 1/2 teaspoon dried oregano, 1/4 teaspoon salt, and 1/4 teaspoon black pepper. Pour dressing over pasta and mix. enjoy!

49. **Vegan Chickpea Salad**: This salad is packed with protein. To make the salad, use 1 can of chickpeas (drained and washed), 1 diced red bell pepper, 1 diced yellow bell pepper, 1 diced cucumber, and 1/4 chopped red onion. cup, 1/4 cup chopped fresh parsley in a large bowl. In a separate bowl, combine 1/4 cup olive oil, 2 tablespoons lemon juice, 1 minced garlic clove, 1/2 teaspoon salt, and 1/4 teaspoon black pepper. Pour dressing over salad and mix. enjoy!

50. **Vegan Lentil Soup**: This soup is hearty and filling. To make the soup, heat 1 tablespoon of the olive oil in a large pot over medium heat. Add 1 chopped onion, 2 chopped carrots, and 2 chopped celery sticks. Cook until the vegetables are soft. Add 2 minced garlic cloves and cook for 1 minute. Add 1 cup dried lentils, 4 cups vegetable broth, 1 can diced tomatoes, 1 teaspoon dried thyme, 1 teaspoon dried oregano, 1/2 teaspoon salt, and 1/4 teaspoon

black pepper. Once it boils, reduce the heat and simmer for about 30 minutes. enjoy!

51. **Vegan Chickpea Salad Sandwich**: This sandwich is a great way to enjoy a protein-packed lunch. To make the sandwich, mash 1 can of chickpeas (drained and washed) with a fork. Add 1/4 cup vegan mayonnaise, 1 tablespoon Dijon mustard, 1 tablespoon nutritional yeast, 1/4 teaspoon salt, and 1/4 teaspoon black pepper. Mix well. Spread the chickpea salad on bread and top with lettuce, tomato, and avocado. Top with another slice of bread and enjoy.

52. **Vegan Quinoa Salad**: This salad is packed with protein and fiber. For the salad, cook 1 cup of quinoa according to package directions. Drain and wash the quinoa. Add diced cucumber, diced red onion, diced red bell pepper, and chopped fresh parsley. In a separate bowl, combine 1/4 cup olive oil, 2 tablespoons lemon juice, 1 minced garlic clove, 1/2 teaspoon salt, and 1/4 teaspoon black pepper. Pour dressing over salad and mix. enjoy!

53. **Vegan Falafel Wrap**: This wrap is the perfect way to enjoy the flavors of the Middle East. For the wrap, spread hummus on a large tortilla. Top with falafel balls, chopped lettuce, diced tomatoes, and diced cucumber. Wrap it in a tortilla and enjoy!

54. **Vegan Chickpea Salad**: This salad is high in protein. To make the salad, use 1 can of chickpeas (drained and washed), 1 diced red bell pepper, 1 diced yellow bell pepper, 1 diced cucumber, and 1/4 chopped red onion. Cup, 1/4 cup chopped fresh parsley in a large bowl. In a separate bowl, combine 1/4 cup olive oil, 2 tablespoons lemon juice, 1 minced garlic clove, 1/2 teaspoon salt, and 1/4 teaspoon black pepper. Pour dressing over salad and mix. Enjoy!

55. **Vegan Lentil Soup**: This soup is hearty and filling. To make the soup, heat 1 tablespoon of the olive oil in a large pot over medium heat. Add 1 chopped onion, 2 chopped carrots, and 2 chopped celery sticks. Cook until the vegetables are soft. Add 2 minced garlic cloves and cook for 1 minute. Add 1 cup dried lentils, 4 cups

vegetable broth, 1 can diced tomatoes, 1 teaspoon dried thyme, 1 teaspoon dried oregano, 1/2 teaspoon salt, and 1/4 teaspoon black pepper. Once it boils, reduce the heat and simmer for about 30 minutes. enjoy!

56. **Vegan Chickpea Salad Sandwich**: This sandwich is a great way to enjoy a protein-packed lunch. To make the sandwich, mash 1 can of chickpeas (drained and washed) with a fork. Add 1/4 cup vegan mayonnaise, 1 tablespoon Dijon mustard, 1 tablespoon nutritional yeast, 1/4 teaspoon salt, and 1/4 teaspoon black pepper. Mix well. Spread the chickpea salad on bread and top with lettuce, tomato, and avocado. Top with another slice of bread and enjoy.

57. **Vegan Quinoa Salad**: This salad is packed with protein and fiber. For the salad, cook 1 cup of quinoa according to package directions. Drain and wash the quinoa. Add diced cucumber, diced red onion, diced red bell pepper, and chopped fresh parsley. In a separate bowl, combine 1/4 cup olive oil, 2 tablespoons lemon juice, 1 minced garlic clove, 1/2 teaspoon salt, and 1/4 teaspoon black pepper. Pour dressing over salad and mix. enjoy!

58. **Vegan Buffalo Cauliflower Wraps**: These wraps are a great way to enjoy the flavor of buffalo sauce. To prepare the wraps, preheat the oven to 200°C. Cut 1 cauliflower into florets. In a large bowl, combine 1/4 cup hot sauce, 2 tablespoons melted vegan butter, 1 tablespoon apple cider vinegar, 1/2 teaspoon garlic powder, and 1/4 teaspoon salt. Add the cauliflower florets and mix. Spread the cauliflower on a baking sheet and bake for 20 minutes. To assemble wraps, spread vegan ranch dressing onto a large tortilla. Top with roasted cauliflower, chopped lettuce, and diced tomatoes. Wrap it in a tortilla and enjoy!

59. **Vegan Chickpea Noodle Soup**: This soup is hearty and filling. To make the soup, heat 1 tablespoon of the olive oil in a large pot over medium heat. Add 1 chopped onion, 2 chopped carrots, and 2 chopped celery sticks. Cook until the vegetables are soft.

Add 2 minced garlic cloves and cook for 1 minute. Add 1 can of chickpeas (drained and washed), 4 cups of vegetable broth, 1 cup of cooked pasta, 1 teaspoon of dried thyme, 1/2 teaspoon of salt, and 1/4 teaspoon of black pepper. Once it boils, reduce the heat and simmer for about 30 minutes. enjoy!

60. **Vegan Falafel Salad:** This salad is a great way to enjoy the flavors of the Middle East. To make the salad, combine chopped lettuce, diced tomatoes, diced cucumber, and red onion slices in a large bowl. Add falafel balls and drizzle with tahini dressing. enjoy!

61. **Vegan Chickpea Tuna Melt:** This sandwich is a great way to enjoy a classic tuna melt. To make the sandwich, mash 1 can of chickpeas (drained and washed) with a fork. Add 1/4 cup vegan mayonnaise, 1 tablespoon Dijon mustard, 1 tablespoon nutritional yeast, 1/4 teaspoon salt, and 1/4 teaspoon black pepper. Mix well. Spread the chickpea salad on bread and top with vegan cheese. Bake until the cheese is melted. enjoy!

62. **Vegan Greek Pasta:** This pasta dish is the perfect way to enjoy the flavors of Greece. To prepare pasta, cook 8 ounces of pasta according to package directions. Drain and wash the noodles. Add chopped cucumber, chopped red onion, chopped kalamata olives, and crumbled vegan feta cheese. In a separate bowl, combine 1/4 cup olive oil, 2 tablespoons red wine vinegar, 1 minced garlic clove, 1/2 teaspoon dried oregano, 1/4 teaspoon salt, and 1/4 teaspoon black pepper. Pour dressing over pasta and mix. enjoy!

63. **Vegan Chickpea Salad:** This salad is high in protein. To make the salad, use 1 can of chickpeas (drained and washed), 1 diced red bell pepper, 1 diced yellow bell pepper, 1 diced cucumber, and 1/4 chopped red onion. Cup, 1/4 cup chopped fresh parsley in a large bowl. In a separate bowl, combine 1/4 cup olive oil, 2 tablespoons lemon juice, 1 minced garlic clove, 1/2 teaspoon salt, and 1/4 teaspoon black pepper. Pour dressing over salad and mix. enjoy!

64. **Vegan Lentil Soup:** This soup is hearty and filling. To make

the soup, heat 1 tablespoon of the olive oil in a large pot over medium heat. Add 1 chopped onion, 2 chopped carrots, and 2 chopped celery sticks. Cook until the vegetables are soft. Add 2 minced garlic cloves and cook for 1 minute. Add 1 cup dried lentils, 4 cups vegetable broth, 1 can diced tomatoes, 1 teaspoon dried thyme, 1 teaspoon dried oregano, 1/2 teaspoon salt, and 1/4 teaspoon black pepper. Once it boils, reduce the heat and simmer for about 30 minutes. enjoy!

65. **Vegan Chickpea Salad Sandwich**: This sandwich is a great way to enjoy a protein-packed lunch. To make the sandwich, mash 1 can of chickpeas (drained and washed) with a fork. Add 1/4 cup vegan mayonnaise, 1 tablespoon Dijon mustard, 1 tablespoon nutritional yeast, 1/4 teaspoon salt, and 1/4 teaspoon black pepper. Mix well. Spread the chickpea salad on bread and top with lettuce, tomato, and avocado. Top with another slice of bread and enjoy.

66. **Vegan Quinoa Salad**: This salad is packed with protein and fiber. For the salad, cook 1 cup of quinoa according to package directions. Drain and wash the quinoa. Add diced cucumber, diced red onion, diced red bell pepper, and chopped fresh parsley. In a separate bowl, combine 1/4 cup olive oil, 2 tablespoons lemon juice, 1 minced garlic clove, 1/2 teaspoon salt, and 1/4 teaspoon black pepper. Pour dressing over salad and mix. enjoy!

67. **Vegan Buffalo Cauliflower Wraps**: These wraps are a great way to enjoy the flavor of buffalo sauce. To prepare the wraps, preheat the oven to 200°C. Cut 1 cauliflower into florets. In a large bowl, combine 1/4 cup hot sauce, 2 tablespoons melted vegan butter, 1 tablespoon apple cider vinegar, 1/2 teaspoon garlic powder, and 1/4 teaspoon salt. Add the cauliflower florets and mix. Spread the cauliflower on a baking sheet and bake for 20 minutes. To assemble wraps, spread vegan ranch dressing onto a large tortilla. Top with roasted cauliflower, chopped lettuce, and diced tomatoes. Wrap it in a tortilla and enjoy!

68. **Vegan Chickpea Noodle Soup**: This soup is hearty and filling. To make the soup, heat 1 tablespoon of the olive oil in a large pot over medium heat. Add 1 chopped onion, 2 chopped carrots, and 2 chopped celery sticks. Cook until the vegetables are soft. Add 2 minced garlic cloves and cook for 1 minute. Add 1 can of chickpeas (drained and washed), 4 cups of vegetable broth, 1 cup of cooked pasta, 1 teaspoon of dried thyme, 1/2 teaspoon of salt, and 1/4 teaspoon of black pepper. Once it boils, reduce the heat and simmer for about 30 minutes. enjoy!

69. **Vegan Falafel Salad**: This salad is a great way to enjoy the flavors of the Middle East. To make the salad, combine chopped lettuce, diced tomatoes, diced cucumber, and red onion slices in a large bowl. Add falafel balls and drizzle with tahini dressing. enjoy!

70. **Vegan Chickpea Tuna Melt**: This sandwich is a great way to enjoy a classic tuna melt. To make the sandwich, mash 1 can of chickpeas (drained and washed) with a fork. Add 1/4 cup vegan mayonnaise, 1 tablespoon Dijon mustard, 1 tablespoon nutritional yeast, 1/4 teaspoon salt, and 1/4 teaspoon black pepper. Mix well. Spread the chickpea salad on bread and top with vegan cheese. Bake until the cheese is melted. enjoy!

71. **Vegan Greek Pasta**: This pasta dish is the perfect way to enjoy the flavors of Greece. To prepare pasta, cook 8 ounces of pasta according to package directions. Drain and wash the noodles. Add chopped cucumber, chopped red onion, chopped kalamata olives, and crumbled vegan feta cheese. In a separate bowl, combine 1/4 cup olive oil, 2 tablespoons red wine vinegar, 1 minced garlic clove, 1/2 teaspoon dried oregano, 1/4 teaspoon salt, and 1/4 teaspoon black pepper. Pour dressing over pasta and mix. enjoy!

72. **Vegan Chickpea Salad**: This salad is rich in protein. To make the salad, use 1 can of chickpeas (drained and washed), 1 diced red bell pepper, 1 diced yellow bell pepper, 1 diced cucumber, and 1/4 chopped red onion. cup, 1/4 cup chopped fresh parsley in a large

bowl. In a separate bowl, combine 1/4 cup olive oil, 2 tablespoons lemon juice, 1 minced garlic clove, 1/2 teaspoon salt, and 1/4 teaspoon black pepper. Pour dressing over salad and mix. enjoy!

73. **Vegan Lentil Soup**: This soup is hearty and filling. To make the soup, heat 1 tablespoon of the olive oil in a large pot over medium heat. Add 1 chopped onion, 2 chopped carrots, and 2 chopped celery sticks. Cook until the vegetables are soft. Add 2 minced garlic cloves and cook for 1 minute. Add 1 cup dried lentils, 4 cups vegetable broth, 1 can diced tomatoes, 1 teaspoon dried thyme, 1 teaspoon dried oregano, 1/2 teaspoon salt, and 1/4 teaspoon black pepper. Once it boils, reduce the heat and simmer for about 30 minutes. enjoy!

74. **Vegan Chickpea Salad Sandwich**: This sandwich is a great way to enjoy a protein-packed lunch. To make the sandwich, mash 1 can of chickpeas (drained and washed) with a fork. Add 1/4 cup vegan mayonnaise, 1 tablespoon Dijon mustard, 1 tablespoon nutritional yeast, 1/4 teaspoon salt, and 1/4 teaspoon black pepper. Mix well. Spread the chickpea salad on bread and top with lettuce, tomato, and avocado. Top with another slice of bread and enjoy.

75. **Vegan Quinoa Chili**: This chili is rich in protein and fiber. To prepare chili peppers, heat 1 tablespoon olive oil in a large pot over medium-high heat. Add 1 chopped onion, 2 chopped carrots, and 2 chopped celery sticks. Cook until the vegetables are soft. Add 2 minced garlic cloves and cook for 1 minute. 1 can diced tomatoes, 1 can tomato sauce, 1 can kidney beans (drained and washed), 1 can black beans (drained and washed), 1 cup quinoa, 2 cups vegetable broth, 1 tablespoon chili powder, Add 1 teaspoon cumin powder. 1/2 teaspoon salt and 1/4 teaspoon black pepper. Once it boils, reduce the heat and simmer for about 30 minutes. enjoy!

76. **Vegan Chickpea Salad**: This salad is packed with protein. To make the salad, use 1 can of chickpeas (drained and washed), 1 diced red bell pepper, 1 diced yellow bell pepper, 1 diced cucumber,

and 1/4 chopped red onion. cup, 1/4 cup chopped fresh parsley in a large bowl. In a separate bowl, combine 1/4 cup olive oil, 2 tablespoons lemon juice, 1 minced garlic clove, 1/2 teaspoon salt, and 1/4 teaspoon black pepper. Pour dressing over salad and mix. enjoy!

77. **Vegan Lentil Soup**: This soup is hearty and filling. To make the soup, heat 1 tablespoon of the olive oil in a large pot over medium heat. Add 1 chopped onion, 2 chopped carrots, and 2 chopped celery sticks. Cook until the vegetables are soft. Add 2 minced garlic cloves and cook for 1 minute. Add 1 cup dried lentils, 4 cups vegetable broth, 1 can diced tomatoes, 1 teaspoon dried thyme, 1 teaspoon dried oregano, 1/2 teaspoon salt, and 1/4 teaspoon black pepper. Once it boils, reduce the heat and simmer for about 30 minutes. enjoy!

78. **Vegan Chickpea Salad Sandwich**: This sandwich is a great way to enjoy a protein-packed lunch. To make the sandwich, mash 1 can of chickpeas (drained and washed) with a fork. Add 1/4 cup vegan mayonnaise, 1 tablespoon Dijon mustard, 1 tablespoon nutritional yeast, 1/4 teaspoon salt, and 1/4 teaspoon black pepper. Mix well. Spread the chickpea salad on bread and top with lettuce, tomato, and avocado. Top with another slice of bread and enjoy.

79. **Vegan Quinoa Salad**: This salad is packed with protein and fiber. For the salad, cook 1 cup of quinoa according to package directions. Drain and wash the quinoa. Add diced cucumber, diced red onion, diced red bell pepper, and chopped fresh parsley. In a separate bowl, combine 1/4 cup olive oil, 2 tablespoons lemon juice, 1 minced garlic clove, 1/2 teaspoon salt, and 1/4 teaspoon black pepper. Pour dressing over salad and mix. enjoy!

80. **Vegan Buffalo Cauliflower Wraps**: These wraps are a great way to enjoy the flavor of buffalo sauce. To prepare the wraps, preheat the oven to 200°C. Cut 1 cauliflower into florets. In a large bowl, combine 1/4 cup hot sauce, 2 tablespoons melted vegan butter, 1

tablespoon apple cider vinegar, 1/2 teaspoon garlic powder, and 1/4 teaspoon salt. Add the cauliflower florets and mix. Spread the cauliflower on a baking sheet and bake for 20 minutes. To assemble wraps, spread vegan ranch dressing onto a large tortilla. Top with roasted cauliflower, chopped lettuce, and diced tomatoes. Wrap it in a tortilla and enjoy!

81. **Spicy Buffalo Chickpea Wraps**: These wraps are a great way to enjoy the flavor of buffalo sauce. To prepare the wraps, combine 1 can chickpeas (drained and rinsed), 1/4 cup hot sauce, 2 tablespoons melted vegan butter, 1/2 teaspoon garlic powder, and 1/4 teaspoon salt in a large bowl. Mash the chickpeas with a fork until they crumble. Spread hummus onto a large tortilla. Top with chickpea mixture, chopped lettuce, and diced tomatoes. Wrap it in a tortilla and enjoy.

82. **Vegan Greek Salad**: This salad is a great way to enjoy the flavors of Greece. For the salad, cut lettuce, tomato, cucumber, and red onion. Add sliced kalamata olives and crumbled vegan feta cheese. Drizzle with olive oil and red wine vinegar. Mix well and enjoy.

83. **Vegan Lentil Soup**: This soup is hearty and filling. To make the soup, heat 1 tablespoon of the olive oil in a large pot over medium heat. Add 1 chopped onion, 2 chopped carrots, and 2 chopped celery sticks. Cook until the vegetables are soft. Add 2 minced garlic cloves and cook for 1 minute. Add 1 cup dried lentils, 4 cups vegetable broth, 1 can diced tomatoes, 1 teaspoon dried thyme, 1 teaspoon dried oregano, 1/2 teaspoon salt, and 1/4 teaspoon black pepper. Once it boils, reduce the heat and simmer for about 30 minutes. Enjoy

84. **Vegan Chickpea Salad Sandwich**: This sandwich is a great way to enjoy a protein-packed lunch. To make the sandwich, mash 1 can of chickpeas (drained and washed) with a fork. Add 1/4 cup vegan mayonnaise, 1 tablespoon Dijon mustard, 1 tablespoon nutritional yeast, 1/4 teaspoon salt, and 1/4 teaspoon black

pepper. Mix well. Spread the chickpea salad on bread and top with lettuce, tomato, and avocado. Place another slice of bread on top and enjoy .

85. **Vegan Quinoa Salad**: This salad is packed with protein and fiber. For the salad, cook 1 cup of quinoa according to package directions. Drain and wash the quinoa. Add diced cucumber, diced red onion, diced red bell pepper, and chopped fresh parsley. In a separate bowl, combine 1/4 cup olive oil, 2 tablespoons lemon juice, 1 minced garlic clove, 1/2 teaspoon salt, and 1/4 teaspoon black pepper. Pour dressing over salad and mix. Enjoy

86. **Vegan Buffalo Cauliflower Wraps**: These wraps are a great way to enjoy the flavor of buffalo sauce. To prepare the wraps, preheat the oven to 200°C. Cut 1 cauliflower into florets. In a large bowl, combine 1/4 cup hot sauce, 2 tablespoons melted vegan butter, 1 tablespoon apple cider vinegar, 1/2 teaspoon garlic powder, and 1/4 teaspoon salt. Add the cauliflower florets and mix. Spread the cauliflower on a baking sheet and bake for 20 minutes. To assemble wraps, spread vegan ranch dressing onto a large tortilla. Top with roasted cauliflower, chopped lettuce, and diced tomatoes. Serve wrapped in a tortilla.

87. **Vegan Chickpea Noodle Soup**: This soup is hearty and filling. To make the soup, heat 1 tablespoon of the olive oil in a large pot over medium heat. Add 1 chopped onion, 2 chopped carrots, and 2 chopped celery sticks. Cook until the vegetables are soft. Add 2 minced garlic cloves and cook for 1 minute. Add 1 can of chickpeas (drained and washed), 4 cups of vegetable broth, 1 cup of cooked pasta, 1 teaspoon of dried thyme, 1/2 teaspoon of salt, and 1/4 teaspoon of black pepper. Once it boils, reduce the heat and simmer for about 30 minutes. Enjoy

88. **Spicy Buffalo Chickpea Wraps**: These wraps are a great way to enjoy the flavor of buffalo sauce. To prepare the wraps, combine 1 can chickpeas (drained and rinsed), 1/4 cup hot sauce, 2 tablespoons melted vegan butter, 1/2 teaspoon garlic powder, and

1/4 teaspoon salt in a large bowl. Mash the chickpeas with a fork until they crumble. Spread hummus onto a large tortilla. Top with chickpea mixture, chopped lettuce, and diced tomatoes. Wrap it in a tortilla and enjoy.

89. **Vegan Greek Salad**: This salad is a great way to enjoy the flavors of Greece. For the salad, cut lettuce, tomato, cucumber, and red onion. Add sliced kalamata olives and crumbled vegan feta cheese. Drizzle with olive oil and red wine vinegar. Mix well and enjoy.

90. **Vegan Lentil Soup**: This soup is hearty and filling. To make the soup, heat 1 tablespoon of the olive oil in a large pot over medium heat. Add 1 chopped onion, 2 chopped carrots, and 2 chopped celery sticks. Cook until the vegetables are soft. Add 2 minced garlic cloves and cook for 1 minute. Add 1 cup dried lentils, 4 cups vegetable broth, 1 can diced tomatoes, 1 teaspoon dried thyme, 1 teaspoon dried oregano, 1/2 teaspoon salt, and 1/4 teaspoon black pepper. Once it boils, reduce the heat and simmer for about 30 minutes. Enjoy

91. **Vegan Chickpea Salad Sandwich**: This sandwich is a great way to enjoy a protein-packed lunch. To make the sandwich, mash 1 can of chickpeas (drained and washed) with a fork. Add 1/4 cup vegan mayonnaise, 1 tablespoon Dijon mustard, 1 tablespoon nutritional yeast, 1/4 teaspoon salt, and 1/4 teaspoon black pepper. Mix well. Spread the chickpea salad on bread and top with lettuce, tomato, and avocado. Top with another slice of bread and enjoy.

92. **Vegan Quinoa Salad**: This salad is packed with protein and fiber. For the salad, cook 1 cup of quinoa according to package directions. Drain and wash the quinoa. Add diced cucumber, diced red onion, diced red bell pepper, and chopped fresh parsley. In a separate bowl, combine 1/4 cup olive oil, 2 tablespoons lemon juice, 1 minced garlic clove, 1/2 teaspoon salt, and 1/4 teaspoon black pepper. Pour dressing over salad and mix. enjoy!

93. **Vegan Buffalo Cauliflower Wraps**: These wraps are a great way to enjoy the flavor of buffalo sauce. To prepare the wraps, preheat the oven to 200°C. Cut 1 cauliflower into florets. In a large bowl, combine 1/4 cup hot sauce, 2 tablespoons melted vegan butter, 1 tablespoon apple cider vinegar, 1/2 teaspoon garlic powder, and 1/4 teaspoon salt. Add the cauliflower florets and mix. Spread the cauliflower on a baking sheet and bake for 20 minutes. To assemble wraps, spread vegan ranch dressing onto a large tortilla. Top with roasted cauliflower, chopped lettuce, and diced tomatoes. Wrap it in a tortilla and enjoy.

94. **Vegan Chickpea Noodle Soup**: This soup is hearty and filling. To make the soup, heat 1 tablespoon of the olive oil in a large pot over medium heat. Add 1 chopped onion, 2 chopped carrots, and 2 chopped celery sticks. Cook until the vegetables are soft. Add 2 minced garlic cloves and cook for 1 minute. Add 1 can of chickpeas (drained and washed), 4 cups of vegetable broth, 1 cup of cooked pasta, 1 teaspoon of dried thyme, 1/2 teaspoon of salt, and 1/4 teaspoon of black pepper. Once it boils, reduce the heat and simmer for about 30 minutes. Enjoy

95. **Vegan Falafel Salad**: This salad is a great way to enjoy the flavors of the Middle East. To make the salad, combine chopped lettuce, diced tomatoes, diced cucumber, and red onion slices in a large bowl. Add falafel balls and drizzle with tahini dressing. Enjoy

96. **Spicy Buffalo Chickpea Wraps**: These wraps are a great way to enjoy the flavor of buffalo sauce. To prepare the wraps, combine 1 can chickpeas (drained and rinsed), 1/4 cup hot sauce, 2 tablespoons melted vegan butter, 1/2 teaspoon garlic powder, and 1/4 teaspoon salt in a large bowl. Mash the chickpeas with a fork until they crumble. Spread hummus onto a large tortilla. Top with chickpea mixture, chopped lettuce, and diced tomatoes. Roll up a tortilla and enjoy

97. **Vegan Greek Salad**: This salad is a great way to enjoy the

flavors of Greece. For the salad, cut lettuce, tomato, cucumber, and red onion. Add sliced kalamata olives and crumbled vegan feta cheese. Drizzle with olive oil and red wine vinegar. Mix well and enjoy.

98. **Vegan Lentil Soup**: This soup is hearty and filling. To make the soup, heat 1 tablespoon of the olive oil in a large pot over medium heat. Add 1 chopped onion, 2 chopped carrots, and 2 chopped celery sticks. Cook until the vegetables are soft. Add 2 minced garlic cloves and cook for 1 minute. Add 1 cup dried lentils, 4 cups vegetable broth, 1 can diced tomatoes, 1 teaspoon dried thyme, 1 teaspoon dried oregano, 1/2 teaspoon salt, and 1/4 teaspoon black pepper. Once it boils, reduce the heat and simmer for about 30 minutes. Enjoy

99. **Vegan Chickpea Salad Sandwich**: This sandwich is a great way to enjoy a protein-packed lunch. To make the sandwich, mash 1 can of chickpeas (drained and washed) with a fork. Add 1/4 cup vegan mayonnaise, 1 tablespoon Dijon mustard, 1 tablespoon nutritional yeast, 1/4 teaspoon salt, and 1/4 teaspoon black pepper. Mix well. Spread the chickpea salad on bread and top with lettuce, tomato, and avocado. Place another slice of bread on top and enjoy

100. **Vegan Quinoa Salad**: This salad is packed with protein and fiber. For the salad, cook 1 cup of quinoa according to package directions. Drain and wash the quinoa. Add diced cucumber, diced red onion, diced red bell pepper, and chopped fresh parsley. In a separate bowl, combine 1/4 cup olive oil, 2 tablespoons lemon juice, 1 minced garlic clove, 1/2 teaspoon salt, and 1/4 teaspoon black pepper. Pour dressing over salad and mix. Enjoy

101. **Vegan Buffalo Cauliflower Wraps**: These wraps are a great way to enjoy the flavor of buffalo sauce. To prepare the wraps, preheat the oven to 200°C. Cut 1 cauliflower into florets. In a large bowl, combine 1/4 cup hot sauce, 2 tablespoons melted vegan butter, 1 tablespoon apple cider vinegar, 1/2 teaspoon garlic

powder, and 1/4 teaspoon salt. Add the cauliflower florets and mix. Spread the cauliflower on a baking sheet and bake for 20 minutes. To assemble wraps, spread vegan ranch dressing onto a large tortilla. Top with roasted cauliflower, chopped lettuce, and diced tomatoes. Wrap it in a tortilla and enjoy.

102. **Vegan Chickpea Noodle Soup**: This soup is hearty and filling. To make the soup, heat 1 tablespoon of the olive oil in a large pot over medium heat. Add 1 chopped onion, 2 chopped carrots, and 2 chopped celery sticks. Cook until the vegetables are soft. Add 2 minced garlic cloves and cook for 1 minute. Add 1 can of chickpeas (drained and washed), 4 cups of vegetable broth, 1 cup of cooked pasta, 1 teaspoon of dried thyme, 1/2 teaspoon of salt, and 1/4 teaspoon of black pepper. Once it boils, reduce the heat and simmer for about 30 minutes. Enjoy

103. **Vegan Falafel Salad**: This salad is a great way to enjoy the flavors of the Middle East. To make the salad, combine chopped lettuce, diced tomatoes, diced cucumber, and red onion slices in a large bowl. Add falafel balls and drizzle with tahini dressing. Enjoy

104. **Spicy Buffalo Chickpea Wraps**: These wraps are a great way to enjoy the flavor of buffalo sauce. To prepare the wraps, combine 1 can chickpeas (drained and rinsed), 1/4 cup hot sauce, 2 tablespoons melted vegan butter, 1/2 teaspoon garlic powder, and 1/4 teaspoon salt in a large bowl. Mash the chickpeas with a fork until they crumble. Spread hummus onto a large tortilla. Top with chickpea mixture, chopped lettuce, and diced tomatoes. Wrap it in a tortilla and enjoy.

105. **Vegan Greek Salad**: This salad is a great way to enjoy the flavors of Greece. For the salad, cut lettuce, tomato, cucumber, and red onion. Add sliced kalamata olives and crumbled vegan feta cheese. Drizzle with olive oil and red wine vinegar. Mix well and enjoy.

106. **Vegan Lentil Soup**: This soup is hearty and filling. To make

the soup, heat 1 tablespoon of the olive oil in a large pot over medium heat. Add 1 chopped onion, 2 chopped carrots, and 2 chopped celery sticks. Cook until the vegetables are soft. Add 2 minced garlic cloves and cook for 1 minute. Add 1 cup dried lentils, 4 cups vegetable broth, 1 can diced tomatoes, 1 teaspoon dried thyme, 1 teaspoon dried oregano, 1/2 teaspoon salt, and 1/4 teaspoon black pepper. Once it boils, reduce the heat and simmer for about 30 minutes. Enjo1

107. **Vegan Chickpea Salad Sandwich**: This sandwich is a great way to enjoy a protein-packed lunch. To make the sandwich, mash 1 can of chickpeas (drained and washed) with a fork. Add 1/4 cup vegan mayonnaise, 1 tablespoon Dijon mustard, 1 tablespoon nutritional yeast, 1/4 teaspoon salt, and 1/4 teaspoon black pepper. Mix well. Spread the chickpea salad on bread and top with lettuce, tomato, and avocado. Place another slice of bread on top and enjoy

108. **Vegan Quinoa Salad**: This salad is packed with protein and fiber. For the salad, cook 1 cup of quinoa according to package directions. Drain and wash the quinoa. Add diced cucumber, diced red onion, diced red bell pepper, and chopped fresh parsley. In a separate bowl, combine 1/4 cup olive oil, 2 tablespoons lemon juice, 1 minced garlic clove, 1/2 teaspoon salt, and 1/4 teaspoon black pepper. Pour dressing over salad and mix. Enjoy

109. **Vegan Chickpea Salad**: This salad is high in protein. To make the salad, use 1 can of chickpeas (drained and washed), 1 diced red bell pepper, 1 diced yellow bell pepper, 1 diced cucumber, and 1/4 chopped red onion. cup, 1/4 cup chopped fresh parsley in a large bowl. In a separate bowl, combine 1/4 cup olive oil, 2 tablespoons lemon juice, 1 minced garlic clove, 1/2 teaspoon salt, and 1/4 teaspoon black pepper. Pour dressing over salad and mix. Enjoy

110. **Vegan Lentil Soup**: This soup is hearty and filling. To make the soup, heat 1 tablespoon of the olive oil in a large pot over medium heat. Add 1 chopped onion, 2 chopped carrots, and 2

chopped celery sticks. Cook until the vegetables are soft. Add 2 minced garlic cloves and cook for 1 minute. Add 1 cup dried lentils, 4 cups vegetable broth, 1 can diced tomatoes, 1 teaspoon dried thyme, 1 teaspoon dried oregano, 1/2 teaspoon salt, and 1/4 teaspoon black pepper. Once it boils, reduce the heat and simmer for about 30 minutes. Enjoy

111. **Vegan Chickpea Salad Sandwich**: This sandwich is a great way to enjoy a protein-packed lunch. To make the sandwich, mash 1 can of chickpeas (drained and washed) with a fork. Add 1/4 cup vegan mayonnaise, 1 tablespoon Dijon mustard, 1 tablespoon nutritional yeast, 1/4 teaspoon salt, and 1/4 teaspoon black pepper. Mix well. Spread the chickpea salad on bread and top with lettuce, tomato, and avocado. Place another slice of bread on top and enjoy

112. **Vegan Quinoa Salad**: This salad is packed with protein and fiber. For the salad, cook 1 cup of quinoa according to package directions. Drain and wash the quinoa. Add diced cucumber, diced red onion, diced red bell pepper, and chopped fresh parsley. In a separate bowl, combine 1/4 cup olive oil, 2 tablespoons lemon juice, 1 minced garlic clove, 1/2 teaspoon salt, and 1/4 teaspoon black pepper. Pour dressing over salad and mix. Enjoy

113. **Vegan Buffalo Cauliflower Wraps**: These wraps are a great way to enjoy the flavor of buffalo sauce. To prepare the wraps, preheat the oven to 200°C. Cut 1 cauliflower into florets. In a large bowl, combine 1/4 cup hot sauce, 2 tablespoons melted vegan butter, 1 tablespoon apple cider vinegar, 1/2 teaspoon garlic powder, and 1/4 teaspoon salt. Add the cauliflower florets and mix. Spread the cauliflower on a baking sheet and bake for 20 minutes. To assemble wraps, spread vegan ranch dressing onto a large tortilla. Top with roasted cauliflower, chopped lettuce, and diced tomatoes. Roll up a tortilla and enjoy

114. **Vegan Chickpea Noodle Soup**: This soup is hearty and filling. To make the soup, heat 1 tablespoon of the olive oil in a large

pot over medium heat. Add 1 chopped onion, 2 chopped carrots, and 2 chopped celery sticks. Cook until the vegetables are soft. Add 2 minced garlic cloves and cook for 1 minute. Add 1 can of chickpeas (drained and washed), 4 cups of vegetable broth, 1 cup of cooked pasta, 1 teaspoon of dried thyme, 1/2 teaspoon of salt, and 1/4 teaspoon of black pepper. Once it boils, reduce the heat and simmer for about 30 minutes. Enjoy

115. **Vegan Falafel Salad**: This salad is a great way to enjoy the flavors of the Middle East. To make the salad, combine chopped lettuce, diced tomatoes, diced cucumber, and red onion slices in a large bowl. Add falafel balls and drizzle with tahini dressing. Enjoy

CHAPTER 8: DINNER RECIPES

· Delicious and Healthy Dinner Recipes

1. **Vegan Mac and Cheese**: This recipe puts a vegan twist on the classic mac and cheese. To make, you'll need macaroni, vegan butter, flour, almond milk, nutritional yeast, garlic powder, onion powder, salt, and pepper. Cook macaroni according to package directions. Melt the vegan butter in a separate saucepan, add the flour and mix. Add almond milk and stir until mixture thickens. Add nutritional yeast, garlic powder, onion powder, salt, and pepper. Mix well. Combine the boiled macaroni with the sauce and mix thoroughly. Serve hot.

2. **Vegan Chili**: This recipe is perfect for a cozy evening. You will need green beans, black beans, diced tomatoes, tomato sauce, vegetable broth, chili powder, cumin, garlic powder, onion powder, salt, and pepper. Add all ingredients in a pot and heat until boiling.. Reduce heat and simmer for 30 minutes. Serve warm.

3. **Vegan Lentil Soup**: This recipe is hearty and filling. You will need lentils, vegetable stock, diced tomatoes, carrots, celery, onion, garlic, cumin, coriander, salt, and pepper. In a large pot, sauté the onions and garlic until fragrant. Add carrots and celery and cook for a few minutes. Add the lentils, vegetable stock, diced tomatoes, cumin, coriander, salt, and pepper. Once it boils, reduce the heat and simmer for about 30 minutes. Please enjoy hot

4. **Vegan Shepherd's Pie**: This recipe is a vegan version of the classic Shepherd's Pie. You'll need potatoes, vegan butter, almond milk, lentils, vegetable broth, onions, garlic, carrots, peas, corn, thyme, salt, and pepper. Boil the potatoes until soft. Drain and mash with vegan butter and almond milk. In a separate pot, fry onions and garlic until fragrant. Add carrots and cook for a few

minutes. Add lentils, vegetable stock, thyme, salt, and pepper. Simmer for 10 minutes. Cook for an additional 5 minutes after adding peas and corn. Preheat oven to 375°F. Layer the lentil mixture in a baking dish and top with the mashed potatoes. Bake until the top turns golden brown, which should take about 20 minutes.

5. **Vegan Pad Thai**: This recipe is a vegan version of the classic Pad Thai. You will need rice noodles, tofu, garlic, onions, bell peppers, bean sprouts, peanuts, lime, soy sauce, brown sugar, and chili flakes. Cook rice noodles according to package directions. In a separate pot, fry the garlic and onion until fragrant. Cook for a few minutes once the peppers are added. Add tofu and fry until golden brown. Add cooked rice noodles, bean sprouts, peanuts, lime juice, soy sauce, brown sugar, and chili flakes. Mix well. Please enjoy warm.

6. **Vegan Stuffed Peppers with Meat**: This recipe is a delicious and healthy way to enjoy peppers. You'll need bell peppers, quinoa, vegetable stock, onions, garlic, diced tomatoes, corn, black beans, chili powder, cumin, salt, and pepper. Preheat oven to 375°F. Remove the seeds and cut the peppers.. In a separate pot, fry onions and garlic until fragrant. Add quinoa, vegetable stock, diced tomatoes, corn, black beans, chili powder, cumin, salt, and pepper. Mix well. Stuff the peppers with the quinoa mixture. cook for 30 minutes or until the peppers are very soft. Serve hot.

7. **Vegan Lentil Tacos**: This recipe is a vegan version of the classic taco. You will need lentils, vegetable broth, onions, garlic, chili powder, cumin, paprika, salt and pepper. In a large frying pan, sauté the onion and garlic until fragrant. Add lentils, vegetable stock, chili powder, cumin, paprika, salt, and pepper. Cook until the lentils are soft. Place the lentil mixture into taco shells and top with your favorite toppings like lettuce, tomato, and avocado. Enjoy

8. **Vegan Chickpea Curry**: This recipe is a delicious and healthy

way to enjoy chickpeas. You will need chickpeas, coconut milk, onion, garlic, ginger, curry powder, turmeric, cumin, salt, and pepper. In a large frying pan, sauté the onion, garlic, and ginger until fragrant. Add chickpeas, coconut milk, curry powder, turmeric, cumin, salt, and pepper. Cook until the chickpeas are soft. Enjoy warm with rice.

9. **Vegan Mushroom Stroganoff**: This recipe is a vegan version of the classic stroganoff. You will need mushrooms, onions, garlic, vegetable broth, almond milk, flour, Dijon mustard, thyme, salt, and pepper. In a large frying pan, sauté the onion and garlic until fragrant. Add mushrooms and cook until soft. In a separate pot, combine vegetable broth, almond milk, flour, Dijon mustard, thyme, salt, and pepper. Add the sauce to the mushrooms and mix well. Enjoy warm with pasta or rice. Enjoy

10. **Vegan Sweet Potato Chili with Black Beans**: This recipe is perfect for a cozy night in. You'll need sweet potatoes, black beans, diced tomatoes, vegetable broth, onions, garlic, chili powder, cumin, salt, and pepper. In a large pot, sauté the onions and garlic until fragrant. Add sweet potatoes, black beans, diced tomatoes, vegetable stock, chili powder, cumin, salt, and pepper. Once it boils, reduce the heat and simmer for about 30 minutes. Serve hot.

11. **Vegan Mushroom Risotto**: This recipe is a vegan version of the classic risotto. You will need mushrooms, vegetable broth, onions, garlic, arborio rice, white wine, nutritional yeast, thyme, salt and pepper. In a large frying pan, sauté the onion and garlic until fragrant. Add mushrooms and cook until soft. After adding the arborio rice, cook it for a few minutes. Add the white wine and simmer until the liquid evaporates. Add vegetable broth, nutritional yeast, thyme, salt, and pepper. Cook until the rice is soft. Serve hot.

12. **Vegan Lentil Bread**: This recipe is a vegan version of the classic meatloaf. You will need lentils, vegetable broth, onions, garlic,

oats, flaxseed meal, tomato paste, soy sauce, thyme, salt and pepper. Preheat oven to 375°F. In a large bowl, combine lentils, vegetable stock, onion, garlic, oats, flaxseed meal, tomato paste, soy sauce, thyme, salt, and pepper. Transfer the mixture to a loaf pan. Bake for 45 minutes or until golden brown on top. Please enjoy warm.

13. **Vegan Mushroom Risotto**: This recipe is a vegan version of the classic risotto. You will need mushrooms, vegetable broth, onions, garlic, arborio rice, white wine, nutritional yeast, thyme, salt and pepper. In a large frying pan, sauté the onion and garlic until fragrant. Add mushrooms and cook until soft. After adding the arborio rice, cook it for a few minutes. Add the white wine and simmer until the liquid evaporates. Add vegetable broth, nutritional yeast, thyme, salt, and pepper. Cook until the rice is soft. Serve warm.

14. **Vegan Chickpea Salad**: This recipe is perfect for a quick and easy dinner. You will need chickpeas, cucumbers, cherry tomatoes, red onions, parsley, lemon juice, olive oil, salt, and pepper. In a large bowl, combine chickpeas, cucumber, cherry tomatoes, red onion, and parsley. In a separate bowl, combine lemon juice, olive oil, salt, and pepper. After pouring the dressing, give the salad a good mix.

15. **Vegan Stuffed Acorn Squash**: This recipe is a delicious and healthy way to enjoy acorn squash. You'll need acorn squash, quinoa, vegetable stock, onions, garlic, kale, dried cranberries, pecans, thyme, salt, and pepper. Preheat oven to 375°F. Divide the acorn squash in half and extract the seeds. In a separate pot, fry onions and garlic until fragrant. Add quinoa, vegetable stock, kale, dried cranberries, pecans, thyme, salt, and pepper. Mix well. Stuff the acorn squash with the quinoa mixture. Bake for 45 minutes or until squash is tender. Please enjoy hot

16. **Vegan Lentil Shepherd's Pie**: This recipe is a vegan version

of the classic Shepherd's Pie. You'll need potatoes, vegan butter, almond milk, lentils, vegetable broth, onions, garlic, carrots, peas, corn, thyme, salt, and pepper. Boil the potatoes until soft. Drain and mash with vegan butter and almond milk. In a separate pot, fry onions and garlic until fragrant. Add carrots and cook for a few minutes. Add lentils, vegetable stock, thyme, salt, and pepper. Simmer for 10 minutes. Cook for an additional 5 minutes after adding peas and corn. Preheat oven to 375°F. Layer the lentil mixture in a baking dish and top with the mashed potatoes. Bake until the top turns golden brown, which should take about 20 minutes. Serve hot.

17. **Vegan Baked Ziti**: This recipe is a vegan version of the classic baked ziti. You will need ziti noodles, vegan sausage, onions, garlic, tomato sauce, almond milk, nutritional yeast, salt, and pepper. Cook ziti noodles according to package directions. In a separate pot, fry onions and garlic until fragrant. Add the vegan sausage and fry until brown. Add tomato sauce, almond milk, nutritional yeast, salt, and pepper. Mix well. Add the boiled ziti noodles to the sauce and stir well. Preheat oven to 375°F. Transfer the mixture to a baking dish. Bake for 20 minutes or until golden brown on top. Serve warm.

18. **Vegan Stuffed Shells**: This recipe is a delicious and healthy way to enjoy stuffed shells. You'll need jumbo pasta shells, vegan ricotta, spinach, garlic, onions, tomato sauce, almond milk, nutritional yeast, salt, and pepper. Cook jumbo noodle shells according to package directions. In a separate pot, fry onions and garlic until fragrant. Add spinach and cook until wilted. In a large bowl, combine vegan ricotta, spinach, almond milk, nutritional yeast, salt, and pepper. Fill jumbo pasta shells with ricotta mixture. Preheat oven to 375°F. Place the stuffed mussels in a baking dish. Pour the tomato sauce over the bowl. Bake until the top turns golden brown, which should take about 20 minutes. Serve warm.

19. **Vegan Mushroom Stroganoff**: This recipe is a vegan version of

the classic stroganoff. You will need mushrooms, onions, garlic, vegetable broth, almond milk, flour, Dijon mustard, thyme, salt, and pepper. In a large frying pan, sauté the onion and garlic until fragrant. Add mushrooms and cook until soft. In a separate pot, combine vegetable broth, almond milk, flour, Dijon mustard, thyme, salt, and pepper. Add the sauce to the mushrooms and mix well. Enjoy warm with pasta or rice. Enjoy

20. **Vegan Shepherd's Pie**: This recipe is a vegan version of the classic Shepherd's Pie. You'll need potatoes, vegan butter, almond milk, lentils, vegetable broth, onions, garlic, carrots, peas, corn, thyme, salt, and pepper. Boil the potatoes until soft. Drain and mash with vegan butter and almond milk. In a separate pot, fry onions and garlic until fragrant. Add carrots and cook for a few minutes. Add lentils, vegetable stock, thyme, salt, and pepper. Simmer for 10 minutes. Cook for an additional 5 minutes after adding peas and corn. Preheat oven to 375°F. Layer the lentil mixture in a baking dish and top with the mashed potatoes. Bake until the top turns golden brown, which should take about 20 minutes. Serve warm.

21. **Vegan Lentil Soup with Spinach**: This recipe is a healthy and hearty soup perfect for cold winter nights. You will need lentils, vegetable broth, onions, garlic, carrots, celery, spinach, thyme, salt and pepper. In a large pot, sauté the onions and garlic until fragrant. Add carrots and celery and cook for a few minutes. Add lentils, vegetable stock, thyme, salt, and pepper. Once it boils, reduce the heat and simmer for about 30 minutes. Add spinach and cook for another 5 minutes. Serve hot.

22. **Vegan Mushroom Stew**: This recipe is a flavorful and healthy way to enjoy mushrooms. You will need mushrooms, onions, garlic, vegetable broth, almond milk, flour, thyme, salt and pepper. In a large frying pan, sauté the onion and garlic until fragrant. Add mushrooms and cook until soft. In a separate pot, combine vegetable broth, almond milk, flour, thyme, salt, and pepper. Add the sauce to the mushrooms and mix well. Enjoy warm with pasta

or rice. Enjoy

23. **Vegan Curry with Chickpeas and Vegetables**: This recipe is a delicious and healthy way to enjoy chickpeas and vegetables. You will need chickpeas, onions, garlic, ginger, curry powder, turmeric, cumin, salt, pepper, cauliflower, carrots, and peas. In a large frying pan, sauté the onion, garlic, and ginger until fragrant. Add curry powder, turmeric, cumin, salt, and pepper. Add chickpeas, cauliflower, carrots, and peas. Cook until the vegetables are soft. Enjoy warm with rice or naan. Enjoy

24. **Vegan Tofu Skillet**: This recipe is a quick and easy dinner option. You will need tofu, broccoli, bell pepper, onion, garlic, soy sauce, rice vinegar, maple syrup, cornstarch, salt, and pepper. In a large frying pan, sauté the onion and garlic until fragrant. Add broccoli, bell pepper, and tofu. In a separate bowl, combine soy sauce, rice vinegar, maple syrup, cornstarch, salt, and pepper.

25. **Vegan Crockpot BBQ Tofu**: This recipe is a delicious and easy way to enjoy tofu. You will need tofu, barbecue sauce, soy sauce, garlic powder, onion powder, and black pepper. Cut the tofu into cubes and put them in the pot. In a separate bowl, combine barbecue sauce, soy sauce, garlic powder, onion powder, and black pepper. Pour the sauce over the tofu and mix well. Cook on low heat for 4-6 hours. Serve warm.

26. **Vegan Burger with Black Beans**: This recipe is a vegan version of the classic burger. You will need black beans, onion, garlic, breadcrumbs, cumin, chili powder, salt, and pepper. Mash the black beans with a fork in a big bowl. Add onion, garlic, breadcrumbs, cumin, chili powder, salt, and pepper. Mix well. Form patties from the mixture. Heat a grill pan to medium-high heat before using. Cook the patties for 3 to 4 minutes on each side. Serve hot.

27. **Vegan Lentil Sloppy Joe**: This recipe is a vegan version of the classic Sloppy Joe. You will need lentils, onions, garlic, tomato sauce, ketchup, mustard, brown sugar, apple cider vinegar, chili

powder, salt, and pepper. In a large frying pan, sauté the onion and garlic until fragrant. Add lentils, tomato sauce, ketchup, mustard, brown sugar, apple cider vinegar, chili powder, salt, and pepper. Cook until the lentils are soft. Serve warm on bread and enjoy.

28. **Vegan Chickpea Salad Sandwich**: This recipe is a quick and easy lunch option. You'll need chickpeas, celery, red onion, dill pickles, vegan mayonnaise, Dijon mustard, lemon juice, salt, and pepper, Use a fork to mash the chickpeas in a large bowl. Add celery, red onion, dill pickles, vegan mayonnaise, Dijon mustard, lemon juice, salt, and pepper. Mix well. Serve with chickpea salad on bread.

29. **Vegan Mushroom Spinach Lasagna**: This recipe is a vegan version of the classic lasagna. You will need lasagna noodles, mushrooms, spinach, onions, garlic, tomato sauce, almond milk, nutritional yeast, salt, and pepper. Cook lasagna noodles according to package directions. In a large frying pan, sauté the onion and garlic until fragrant. Add mushrooms and cook until soft. Add spinach and cook until wilted. In a separate bowl, combine tomato sauce, almond milk, nutritional yeast, salt, and pepper. Layer lasagna noodles, mushroom mixture, and tomato sauce mixture in a baking dish. Repeat until all ingredients are used. Bake at 180°C for 20-25 minutes or until golden brown on top. Serve warm

30. **Vegan Lentil Soup with Spinach**: This recipe is a healthy and hearty soup perfect for cold winter nights. You will need lentils, vegetable broth, onions, garlic, carrots, celery, spinach, thyme, salt and pepper. In a large pot, sauté the onions and garlic until fragrant. Add carrots and celery and cook for a few minutes. Add lentils, vegetable stock, thyme, salt, and pepper. Once it boils, reduce the heat and simmer for about 30 minutes. Add spinach and cook for another 5 minutes. Please enjoy hot

31. **Vegan Curry with Chickpeas and Vegetables**: This recipe is a delicious and healthy way to enjoy chickpeas and vegetables.

You will need chickpeas, onions, garlic, ginger, curry powder, turmeric, cumin, salt, pepper, cauliflower, carrots, and peas. In a large frying pan, sauté the onion, garlic, and ginger until fragrant. Add curry powder, turmeric, cumin, salt, and pepper. Add chickpeas, cauliflower, carrots, and peas. Cook until the vegetables are soft. Enjoy warm with rice or naan. Enjoy

32. **Vegan Tofu Skillet**: This recipe is a quick and easy dinner option. You will need tofu, broccoli, bell pepper, onion, garlic, soy sauce, rice vinegar, maple syrup, cornstarch, salt, and pepper. In a large frying pan, sauté the onion and garlic until fragrant. Add broccoli, bell pepper, and tofu. In a separate bowl, combine soy sauce, rice vinegar, maple syrup, cornstarch, salt, and pepper. Pour the sauce into the pot and mix it well. Cook until the vegetables are soft. Enjoy with hot rice or noodles. enjoy!

33. **Vegan Lentil and Vegetable Stir-Fry**: This recipe is a quick and easy dinner option. You will need lentils, broccoli, bell peppers, onions, garlic, soy sauce, rice vinegar, maple syrup, cornstarch, salt, and pepper. In a large frying pan, sauté the onion and garlic until fragrant. Add broccoli, peppers, and lentils. In a separate bowl, combine soy sauce, rice vinegar, maple syrup, cornstarch, salt, and pepper. Add the sauce to the pot and mix well. Cook until the vegetables are soft. Enjoy with hot rice or noodles. Enjoy

34. **Vegan Curry with Chickpeas and Spinach**: This recipe is a flavorful and healthy way to enjoy chickpeas and spinach. You will need chickpeas, onions, garlic, ginger, curry powder, turmeric, cumin, salt, pepper, and spinach. In a large frying pan, sauté the onion, garlic, and ginger until fragrant. Add curry powder, turmeric, cumin, salt, and pepper. Add chickpeas and spinach. Cook until spinach wilts. Enjoy warm with rice or naan. Enjoy

35. **Vegan Shepherd's Pie with Mushrooms and Lentils**: This recipe is a vegan version of the classic Shepherd's Pie. You'll need potatoes, vegan butter, almond milk, lentils, vegetable broth,

onions, garlic, mushrooms, carrots, peas, thyme, salt, and pepper. Boil the potatoes until soft. Drain and mash with vegan butter and almond milk. In a separate pot, fry onions and garlic until fragrant. Add mushrooms and cook until soft. Add carrots and cook for a few minutes. Add lentils, vegetable stock, thyme, salt, and pepper. Simmer for 10 minutes. Cook for an additional 5 minutes after adding peas and corn. Preheat oven to 375°F. Layer the lentil mixture in a baking dish and top with the mashed potatoes. Bake until the top turns golden brown, which should take about 20 minutes. Serve warm.

36. **Vegan Tofu and Vegetable Stir-Fry**: This recipe is a quick and easy dinner option. You will need tofu, broccoli, bell pepper, onion, garlic, soy sauce, rice vinegar, maple syrup, cornstarch, salt, and pepper. In a large frying pan, sauté the onion and garlic until fragrant. Add broccoli, bell pepper, and tofu. In a separate bowl, combine soy sauce, rice vinegar, maple syrup, cornstarch, salt, and pepper. Add the sauce to the pot and mix well. Cook until the vegetables are soft. Enjoy with hot rice or noodles. Enjoy

37. **Vegan Lentil and Vegetable Soup**: This recipe is a healthy and hearty soup perfect for cold winter nights. You will need lentils, vegetable broth, onions, garlic, carrots, celery, zucchini, thyme, salt and pepper. In a large pot, sauté the onions and garlic until fragrant. Cook for a few minutes after adding carrots, celery, and zucchini. Add lentils, vegetable stock, thyme, salt, and pepper. Once it boils, reduce the heat and simmer for about 30 minutes. Enjoy hot!

38. **Vegan Lentil and Vegetable Stir-Fry**: This recipe is a quick and easy dinner option. You will need lentils, broccoli, bell peppers, onions, garlic, soy sauce, rice vinegar, maple syrup, cornstarch, salt, and pepper. In a large frying pan, sauté the onion and garlic until fragrant. Add broccoli, peppers, and lentils. In a separate bowl, combine soy sauce, rice vinegar, maple syrup, cornstarch, salt, and pepper. Add the sauce to the pot and mix well. Cook until the vegetables are soft. Enjoy with hot rice or noodles. Enjoy

39. **Vegan Curry with Chickpeas and Spinach**: This recipe is a flavorful and healthy way to enjoy chickpeas and spinach. You will need chickpeas, onions, garlic, ginger, curry powder, turmeric, cumin, salt, pepper, and spinach. In a large frying pan, sauté the onion, garlic, and ginger until fragrant. Add curry powder, turmeric, cumin, salt, and pepper. Add chickpeas and spinach. Cook until spinach wilts. Enjoy warm with rice or naan. Enjoy

40. **Vegan Mushroom and Lentil Shepherd's Pie**: This recipe is a vegan take on the classic shepherd's pie. You'll need potatoes, vegan butter, almond milk, lentils, vegetable broth, onions, garlic, mushrooms, carrots, peas, thyme, salt, and pepper. Boil the potatoes until soft. Drain and mash with vegan butter and almond milk. In a separate pot, fry onions and garlic until fragrant. Add mushrooms and cook until soft. Add carrots and cook for a few minutes. Add lentils, vegetable stock, thyme, salt, and pepper. Simmer for 10 minutes Cook for an additional 5 minutes after adding peas and corn. Preheat oven to 375°F. Layer the lentil mixture in a baking dish and top with the mashed potatoes. Bake until the top turns golden brown, which should take about 20 minutes. Serve hot

41. **Vegan Tofu and Vegetable Stir-Fry**: This recipe is a quick and easy dinner option. You will need tofu, broccoli, bell pepper, onion, garlic, soy sauce, rice vinegar, maple syrup, cornstarch, salt, and pepper. In a large frying pan, sauté the onion and garlic until fragrant. Add broccoli, bell pepper, and tofu. In a separate bowl, combine soy sauce, rice vinegar, maple syrup, cornstarch, salt, and pepper. Add the sauce to the pot and mix well. Cook until the vegetables are soft. Enjoy with hot rice or noodles. Enjoy

42. **Vegan Lentil and Vegetable Soup**: This recipe is a healthy and hearty soup perfect for cold winter nights. You will need lentils, vegetable broth, onions, garlic, carrots, celery, zucchini, thyme, salt and pepper. In a large pot, sauté the onions and garlic until fragrant. Cook for a few minutes after adding carrots, celery, and

zucchini. Add lentils, vegetable stock, thyme, salt, and pepper. Once it boils, reduce the heat and simmer for about 30 minutes. Enjoy hot!

43. **Vegan Spaghetti Marinara with Lentil Balls**: This recipe is a vegan version of the classic spaghetti and meatballs. You will need spaghetti, lentils, mushrooms, onions, garlic, Italian seasoning, breadcrumbs, marinara sauce, and nutritional yeast. Boil spaghetti according to package directions. In a food processor, combine lentils, mushrooms, onion, garlic, Italian seasoning, breadcrumbs, and nutritional yeast until well combined. Form balls from the mixture and bake in the oven for 20 minutes. Use a separate pot to warm the marinara sauce. Serve spaghetti with lentil balls and marinara sauce. Enjoy

44. **Vegan Butternut Squash Risotto with Leek and Spinach**: This recipe is a comforting and flavorful vegan dinner option. You will need butternut squash, arborio rice, vegetable broth, green onions, spinach, nutritional yeast, and thyme. In a large pot, sauté the green onions until fragrant. Cook the arborio rice for a few minutes.

45. **Vegan Chickpea Sweet Potato Curry**: This recipe is a delicious and healthy way to enjoy chickpeas and sweet potatoes. You will need chickpeas, sweet potatoes, onions, garlic, ginger, curry powder, turmeric, cumin, salt, pepper, and coconut milk. In a large frying pan, sauté the onion, garlic, and ginger until fragrant. Add curry powder, turmeric, cumin, salt, and pepper. Add chickpeas and sweet potatoes. Cook the sweet potatoes until they turn soft. Add coconut milk and mix well. Enjoy warm with rice or naan. Enjoy

46. **Vegan Lentil and Vegetable Stir-Fry**: This recipe is a quick and easy dinner option. You will need lentils, broccoli, bell peppers, onions, garlic, soy sauce, rice vinegar, maple syrup, cornstarch, salt, and pepper. In a large frying pan, sauté the onion and garlic until fragrant. Add broccoli, peppers, and lentils. In a separate

bowl, combine soy sauce, rice vinegar, maple syrup, cornstarch, salt, and pepper. Add the sauce to the pot and mix well. Cook until the vegetables are soft. Enjoy with hot rice or noodles. Enjoy

47. **Vegan Shepherd's Pie with Mushrooms and Lentils**: This recipe is a vegan version of the classic Shepherd's Pie. You'll need potatoes, vegan butter, almond milk, lentils, vegetable broth, onions, garlic, mushrooms, carrots, peas, thyme, salt, and pepper. Boil the potatoes until soft. Drain and mash with vegan butter and almond milk. In a separate pot, fry onions and garlic until fragrant. Add mushrooms and cook until soft. Add carrots and cook for a few minutes. Add lentils, vegetable stock, thyme, salt, and pepper. Simmer for 10 minutes. Cook for an additional 5 minutes after adding peas and corn. Preheat oven to 375°F. Layer the lentil mixture in a baking dish and top with the mashed potatoes. Bake until the top turns golden brown, which should take about 20 minutes. Serve warm

48. **Vegan Lentil and Vegetable Soup**: This recipe is a healthy and hearty soup perfect for cold winter nights. You will need lentils, vegetable broth, onions, garlic, carrots, celery, zucchini, thyme, salt and pepper. In a large pot, sauté the onions and garlic until fragrant. Cook for a few minutes after adding carrots, celery, and zucchini.. Combine lentils, vegetable stock, thyme, salt, and pepper. Once it boils, reduce the heat and simmer for about 30 minutes. Enjoy hot!

49. **Vegan Spaghetti Marinara with Lentil Balls**: This recipe is a vegan take on the classic spaghetti and meatballs. You will need spaghetti, lentils, mushrooms, onions, garlic, Italian seasoning, breadcrumbs, marinara sauce, and nutritional yeast. Boil spaghetti according to package directions. In a food processor, combine lentils, mushrooms, onion, garlic, Italian seasoning, breadcrumbs, and nutritional yeast until well combined. Form balls from the mixture and bake in the oven for 20 minutes. Warm the marinara sauce in a separate pot. Serve spaghetti with lentil balls and marinara sauce. enjoy!

50. **Vegan Spaghetti Marinara with Lentil Balls**: This recipe is a vegan twist on the classic spaghetti and meatballs. You will need spaghetti, lentils, mushrooms, onions, garlic, Italian seasoning, breadcrumbs, marinara sauce, and nutritional yeast. Boil spaghetti according to package directions. In a food processor, combine lentils, mushrooms, onion, garlic, Italian seasoning, breadcrumbs, and nutritional yeast until well combined. Form balls from the mixture and bake in the oven for 20 minutes. Warm the marinara sauce in a separate pot. Serve spaghetti with lentil balls and marinara sauce. Enjoy

51. **Vegan Chickpea Sweet Potato Curry**: This recipe is a delicious and healthy way to enjoy chickpeas and sweet potatoes. You will need chickpeas, sweet potatoes, onions, garlic, ginger, curry powder, turmeric, cumin, salt, pepper, and coconut milk. In a large frying pan, sauté the onion, garlic, and ginger until fragrant. Mix in curry powder, turmeric, cumin, salt, and pepper. Add chickpeas and sweet potatoes. Cook the sweet potatoes until they become tender. Add coconut milk and mix well. Enjoy warm with rice or naan. Enjoy

52. **Vegan Lentil and Vegetable Stir-Fry**: This recipe is a quick and easy dinner option. You will need lentils, broccoli, bell peppers, onions, garlic, soy sauce, rice vinegar, maple syrup, cornstarch, salt, and pepper. In a large frying pan, sauté the onion and garlic until fragrant. Add broccoli, peppers, and lentils. In a separate bowl, combine soy sauce, rice vinegar, maple syrup, cornstarch, salt, and pepper. Add the sauce to the pot and mix well. Cook until the vegetables are soft. Enjoy with hot rice or noodles. Enjoy

53. **Vegan Shepherd's Pie with Mushrooms and Lentils**: This recipe is a vegan version of the classic Shepherd's Pie. You'll need potatoes, vegan butter, almond milk, lentils, vegetable broth, onions, garlic, mushrooms, carrots, peas, thyme, salt, and pepper. Boil the potatoes until soft. Drain and mash with vegan butter and almond milk. In a separate pot, fry onions and garlic until fragrant. Add mushrooms and cook until soft. Add carrots and

cook for a few minutes. Combine lentils, vegetable stock, thyme, salt, and pepper. Simmer for 10 minutes. Add peas and cook for another 5 minutes. Preheat oven to 375°F. Layer the lentil mixture in a baking dish and top with the mashed potatoes. Bake for 20 minutes or until golden brown on top. Serve warm

54. **Vegan Tofu and Vegetable Stir-Fry**: This recipe is a quick and easy dinner option. You will need tofu, broccoli, bell pepper, onion, garlic, soy sauce, rice vinegar, maple syrup, cornstarch, salt, and pepper. In a large frying pan, sauté the onion and garlic until fragrant. Add broccoli, bell pepper, and tofu. In a separate bowl, combine soy sauce, rice vinegar, maple syrup, cornstarch, salt, and pepper. Add the sauce to the pot and mix well. Cook until the vegetables are soft. Enjoy with hot rice or noodles. enjoy!

55. **Vegan Lentil and Vegetable Soup**: This recipe is a healthy and hearty soup perfect for cold winter nights. You will need lentils, vegetable broth, onions, garlic, carrots, celery, zucchini, thyme, salt and pepper. In a large pot, sauté the onions and garlic until fragrant. Cook for a few minutes after adding carrots, celery, and zucchini. Combine lentils, vegetable stock, thyme, salt, and pepper. Once it boils, reduce the heat and simmer for about 30 minutes. Enjoy hot!

56. **Vegan Spicy Peanut Noodles**: This recipe is a quick and easy dinner option. You'll need spaghetti, peanut butter, soy sauce, rice vinegar, maple syrup, garlic, ginger, red pepper flakes, and green onions. Boil spaghetti according to package directions. In a separate bowl, combine peanut butter, soy sauce, rice vinegar, maple syrup, garlic, gingers, and red pepper flakes. Combine the sauce with the spaghetti and mix thoroughly. Top with green onions. Serve hot.

57. **Chickpea and Sweet Potato Vegan Curry**: This recipe is a delicious and healthy way to enjoy chickpeas and sweet potato. You will need chickpeas, sweet potatoes, onions, garlic, ginger, curry powder, turmeric, cumin, salt, pepper, and coconut milk.

In a large frying pan, sauté the onion, garlic, and ginger until fragrant. Add Mix in curry powder, turmeric, cumin, salt, and pepper. Add chickpeas and sweet potatoes. Cook the sweet potatoes until they become tender. Add coconut milk and mix well. Enjoy warm with rice or naan. Enjoy

58. **Vegan Shepherd's Pie with Mushrooms and Lentils**: This recipe is a vegan version of the classic Shepherd's Pie. You'll need potatoes, vegan butter, almond milk, lentils, vegetable broth, onions, garlic, mushrooms, carrots, peas, thyme, salt, and pepper. Boil the potatoes until soft. Drain and mash with vegan butter and almond milk. In a separate pot, fry onions and garlic until fragrant. Add mushrooms and cook until soft. Add carrots and cook for a few minutes. Combine lentils, vegetable stock, thyme, salt, and pepper. Simmer for 10 minutes. Add peas and cook for another 5 minutes. Preheat oven to 375°F. Layer the lentil mixture in a baking dish and top with the mashed potatoes. Bake for 20 minutes or until golden brown on top. Please enjoy hot

59. **Vegan Tofu and Vegetable Stir-Fry**: This recipe is a quick and easy dinner option. You will need tofu, broccoli, bell pepper, onion, garlic, soy sauce, rice vinegar, maple syrup, cornstarch, salt, and pepper. In a large frying pan, sauté the onion and garlic until fragrant. Add broccoli, bell pepper, and tofu. In a separate bowl, combine soy sauce, rice vinegar, maple syrup, cornstarch, salt, and pepper. Add the sauce to the pot and mix well. Cook until the vegetables are soft. Enjoy with hot rice or noodles. enjoy!

60. **Vegan Lentil and Vegetable Soup**: This recipe is a healthy and hearty soup perfect for cold winter nights. You will need lentils, vegetable broth, onions, garlic, carrots, celery, zucchini, thyme, salt and pepper. In a large pot, sauté the onions and garlic until fragrant. Cook for a few minutes after adding carrots, celery, and zucchini. Combine lentils, vegetable stock, thyme, salt, and pepper. Once it boils, reduce the heat and simmer for about 30 minutes. Enjoy hot!

61. **Vegan Spicy Peanut Noodles**: This recipe is a quick and easy dinner option. You'll need spaghetti, peanut butter, soy sauce, rice vinegar, maple syrup, garlic, ginger, red pepper flakes, and green onions. Boil spaghetti according to package directions. In a separate bowl, combine peanut butter, soy sauce, rice vinegar, maple syrup, garlic, gingers, and red pepper flakes. Combine the sauce with the spaghetti and mix thoroughly. Top with green onions. Serve warm.

62. **Chickpea and Sweet Potato Vegan Curry**: This recipe is a delicious and healthy way to enjoy chickpeas and sweet potato. You will need chickpeas, sweet potatoes, onions, garlic, ginger, curry powder, turmeric, cumin, salt, pepper, and coconut milk. In a large frying pan, sauté the onion, garlic, and ginger until fragrant. Mix in curry powder, turmeric, cumin, salt, and pepper. Add chickpeas and sweet potatoes. Cook the sweet potatoes until they become tender. Add coconut milk and mix well. Enjoy warm with rice or naan. Enjoy

63. **Vegan Lentil and Vegetable Soup**: This recipe is a healthy and hearty soup perfect for cold winter nights. You will need lentils, vegetable broth, onions, garlic, carrots, celery, zucchini, thyme, salt and pepper. In a large pot, sauté the onions and garlic until fragrant. Cook for a few minutes after adding carrots, celery, and zucchini. Combine lentils, vegetable stock, thyme, salt, and pepper. Once it boils, reduce the heat and simmer for about 30 minutes. Enjoy hot!

64. **Vegan Butternut Squash Risotto with Leeks and Spinach**: This recipe is a comforting and flavorful vegan dinner option. You will need butternut squash, arborio rice, vegetable broth, green onions, spinach, nutritional yeast, and thyme. In a large pot, sauté the green onions until fragrant. Add the arborio rice and cook for a few minutes. Add vegetable stock and butternut squash. Simmer until the rice is soft. Add spinach, nutritional yeast, and thyme. Mix well. Serve warm

65. **Vegan Butternut Squash Risotto with Leeks and Spinach**: This recipe is a comforting and flavorful vegan dinner option. You will need butternut squash, arborio rice, vegetable broth, green onions, spinach, nutritional yeast, and thyme. In a large pot, sauté the green onions until fragrant. Add the arborio rice and cook for a few minutes. Add vegetable stock and butternut squash. Simmer until the rice is soft. Add spinach, nutritional yeast, and thyme. Mix well. Serve hot.

66. **Vegan Lentil and Vegetable Stew**: This recipe is a hearty and healthy vegan stew perfect for cold winter nights. You will need lentils, vegetable broth, onions, garlic, carrots, celery, zucchini, thyme, salt and pepper. In a large pot, sauté the onions and garlic until fragrant. Cook for a few minutes after adding carrots, celery, and zucchini. Combine lentils, vegetable stock, thyme, salt, and pepper. Once it boils, reduce the heat and simmer for about 30 minutes. Serve warm

67. **Vegan Spicy Peanut Noodles**: This recipe is a quick and easy dinner option. You'll need spaghetti, peanut butter, soy sauce, rice vinegar, maple syrup, garlic, ginger, red pepper flakes, and green onions. Boil spaghetti according to package directions. In a separate bowl, combine peanut butter, soy sauce, rice vinegar, maple syrup, garlic, gingers, and red pepper flakes. Combine the sauce with the spaghetti and mix thoroughly. Top with green onions. Serve hot

68. **Vegan Chickpea Sweet Potato Curry**: This recipe is a delicious and healthy way to enjoy chickpeas and sweet potatoes. You will need chickpeas, sweet potatoes, onions, garlic, ginger, curry powder, turmeric, cumin, salt, pepper, and coconut milk. In a large frying pan, sauté the onion, garlic, and ginger until fragrant. Mix in curry powder, turmeric, cumin, salt, and pepper. Add chickpeas and sweet potatoes. Cook the sweet potatoes until they become tender. Add coconut milk and mix well. Enjoy warm with rice or naan. Enjoy

69. **Vegan Mushroom and Lentil Shepherd's Pie**: This recipe is a vegan version of the classic Shepherd's Pie. You'll need potatoes, vegan butter, almond milk, lentils, vegetable broth, onions, garlic, mushrooms, carrots, peas, thyme, salt, and pepper. Boil the potatoes until soft. Drain and mash with vegan butter and almond milk. In a separate pot, fry onions and garlic until fragrant. Add mushrooms and cook until soft. Add carrots and cook for a few minutes. Combine lentils, vegetable stock, thyme, salt, and pepper. Simmer for 10 minutes. Add peas and cook for another 5 minutes. Preheat oven to 375°F. Layer the lentil mixture in a baking dish and top with the mashed potatoes. Bake for 20 minutes or until golden brown on top. Enjoy hot!

70. **Vegan Tofu and Vegetable Stir-Fry**: This recipe is a quick and easy dinner option. You will need tofu, broccoli, bell pepper, onion, garlic, soy sauce, rice vinegar, maple syrup, cornstarch, salt, and pepper. In a large frying pan, sauté the onion and garlic until fragrant. Add broccoli, bell pepper, and tofu. In a separate bowl, combine soy sauce, rice vinegar, maple syrup, cornstarch, salt, and pepper. Add the sauce to the pot and mix well. Cook until the vegetables are soft. Enjoy with hot rice or noodles. enjoy!

71. **Vegan Lentil and Vegetable Soup**: This recipe is a healthy and hearty soup perfect for cold winter nights. You will need lentils, vegetable broth, onions, garlic, carrots, celery, zucchini, thyme, salt and pepper. In a large pot, sauté the onions and garlic until fragrant. Cook for a few minutes after adding carrots, celery, and zucchini. Combine lentils, vegetable stock, thyme, salt, and pepper. Once it boils, reduce the heat and simmer for about 30 minutes. Enjoy hot!

72. **Vegan Butternut Squash Risotto with Leeks and Spinach**: This recipe is a comforting and flavorful vegan dinner option. You will need butternut squash, arborio rice, vegetable broth, green onions, spinach, nutritional yeast, and thyme. In a large pot, sauté the green onions until fragrant. Add the arborio rice and cook for a few minutes. Add vegetable stock and butternut squash. Simmer

until the rice is soft. Add spinach, nutritional yeast, and thyme. Mix well. Serve hot.

73. **Vegan Lentil and Vegetable Stew**: This recipe is a hearty and healthy vegan stew perfect for cold winter nights. You will need lentils, vegetable broth, onions, garlic, carrots, celery, zucchini, thyme, salt and pepper. In a large pot, sauté the onions and garlic until fragrant. Cook for a few minutes after adding carrots, celery, and zucchini. Combine lentils, vegetable stock, thyme, salt, and pepper. Once it boils, reduce the heat and simmer for about 30 minutes. Serve warm

74. **Vegan Shepherd's Pie with Mushrooms and Lentils**: This recipe is a vegan version of the classic Shepherd's Pie. You'll need potatoes, vegan butter, almond milk, lentils, vegetable broth, onions, garlic, mushrooms, carrots, peas, thyme, salt, and pepper. Boil the potatoes until soft. Drain and mash with vegan butter and almond milk. In a separate pot, fry onions and garlic until fragrant. Add mushrooms and cook until soft. Add carrots and cook for a few minutes. Combine lentils, vegetable stock, thyme, salt, and pepper. Simmer for 10 minutes. Add peas and cook for another 5 minutes. Preheat oven to 375°F. Layer the lentil mixture in a baking dish and top with the mashed potatoes. Bake for 20 minutes or until golden brown on top. Enjoy hot!

75. **Vegan Tofu and Vegetable Stir-Fry**: This recipe is a quick and easy dinner option. You will need tofu, broccoli, bell pepper, onion, garlic, soy sauce, rice vinegar, maple syrup, cornstarch, salt, and pepper. In a large frying pan, sauté the onion and garlic until fragrant. Add broccoli, bell pepper, and tofu. In a separate bowl, combine soy sauce, rice vinegar, maple syrup, cornstarch, salt, and pepper. Add the sauce to the pot and mix well. Cook until the vegetables are soft. Enjoy with hot rice or noodles. enjoy!

76. **Vegan Lentil and Vegetable Stir-Fry**: This recipe is a quick and easy dinner option. You will need lentils, broccoli, bell peppers, onions, garlic, soy sauce, rice vinegar, maple syrup, cornstarch,

salt, and pepper. In a large frying pan, sauté the onion and garlic until fragrant. Add broccoli, peppers, and lentils. In a separate bowl, combine soy sauce, rice vinegar, maple syrup, cornstarch, salt, and pepper. Add the sauce to the pot and mix well. Cook until the vegetables are soft. Enjoy with hot rice or noodles. enjoy!

77. **Vegan Shepherd's Pie with Mushrooms and Lentils**: This recipe is a vegan version of the classic Shepherd's Pie. You'll need potatoes, vegan butter, almond milk, lentils, vegetable broth, onions, garlic, mushrooms, carrots, peas, thyme, salt, and pepper. Boil the potatoes until soft. Drain and mash with vegan butter and almond milk. In a separate pot, fry onions and garlic until fragrant. Add mushrooms and cook until soft. Add carrots and cook for a few minutes. Combine lentils, vegetable stock, thyme, salt, and pepper. Simmer for 10 minutes. Add peas and cook for another 5 minutes. Preheat oven to 375°F. Layer the lentil mixture in a baking dish and top with the mashed potatoes. Bake for 20 minutes or until golden brown on top. Enjoy hot!

78. **Vegan Butternut Squash Risotto with Leeks and Spinach**: This recipe is a comforting and flavorful vegan dinner option. You will need butternut squash, arborio rice, vegetable broth, green onions, spinach, nutritional yeast, and thyme. In a large pot, sauté the green onions until fragrant. Add the arborio rice and cook for a few minutes. Add vegetable stock and butternut squash. Simmer until the rice is soft. Add spinach, nutritional yeast, and thyme. Mix well. Serve warm

79. **Vegan Lentil and Vegetable Stir-Fry**: This recipe is a quick and easy dinner option. You will need lentils, broccoli, bell peppers, onions, garlic, soy sauce, rice vinegar, maple syrup, cornstarch, salt, and pepper. In a large frying pan, sauté the onion and garlic until fragrant. Add broccoli, peppers, and lentils. In a separate bowl, combine soy sauce, rice vinegar, maple syrup, cornstarch, salt, and pepper. Add the sauce to the pot and mix well. Cook until the vegetables are soft. Enjoy with hot rice or noodles. enjoy!

80. **Vegan Shepherd's Pie with Mushrooms and Lentils**: This recipe is a vegan version of the classic Shepherd's Pie. You'll need potatoes, vegan butter, almond milk, lentils, vegetable broth, onions, garlic, mushrooms, carrots, peas, thyme, salt, and pepper. Boil the potatoes until soft. Drain and mash with vegan butter and almond milk. In a separate pot, fry onions and garlic until fragrant. Add mushrooms and cook until soft. Add carrots and cook for a few minutes. Combine lentils, vegetable stock, thyme, salt, and pepper. Simmer for 10 minutes. Add peas and cook for another 5 minutes. Preheat oven to 375°F. Layer the lentil mixture in a baking dish and top with the mashed potatoes. Bake for 20 minutes or until golden brown on top. Enjoy hot!

81. **Vegan Mushroom and Lentil Shepherd's Pie**: This recipe is a vegan version of the classic Shepherd's Pie. You'll need potatoes, vegan butter, almond milk, lentils, vegetable broth, onions, garlic, mushrooms, carrots, peas, thyme, salt, and pepper. Boil the potatoes until soft. Drain and mash with vegan butter and almond milk. In a separate pot, fry onions and garlic until fragrant. Add mushrooms and cook until soft. Add carrots and cook for a few minutes. Combine lentils, vegetable stock, thyme, salt, and pepper. Simmer for 10 minutes. Add peas and cook for another 5 minutes. Preheat oven to 375°F. Layer the lentil mixture in a baking dish and top with the mashed potatoes. Bake for 20 minutes or until golden brown on top. Enjoy hot!

82. **Vegan Tofu and Vegetable Stir-Fry**: This recipe is a quick and easy dinner option. You will need tofu, broccoli, bell pepper, onion, garlic, soy sauce, rice vinegar, maple syrup, cornstarch, salt, and pepper. In a large frying pan, sauté the onion and garlic until fragrant. Add broccoli, bell pepper, and tofu. In a separate bowl, combine soy sauce, rice vinegar, maple syrup, cornstarch, salt, and pepper. Add the sauce to the pot and mix well. Cook until the vegetables are soft. Enjoy with hot rice or noodles. enjoy!

83. **Vegan Lentil and Vegetable Soup**: This recipe is a healthy and hearty soup perfect for cold winter nights. You will need

lentils, vegetable broth, onions, garlic, carrots, celery, zucchini, thyme, salt and pepper. In a large pot, sauté the onions and garlic until fragrant. Cook for a few minutes after adding carrots, celery, and zucchini. Combine lentils, vegetable stock, thyme, salt, and pepper. Once it boils, reduce the heat and simmer for about 30 minutes. Please enjoy hot

84. **Vegan Spicy Peanut Noodles**: This recipe is a quick and easy dinner option. You'll need spaghetti, peanut butter, soy sauce, rice vinegar, maple syrup, garlic, ginger, red pepper flakes, and green onions. Boil spaghetti according to package directions. In a separate bowl, combine peanut butter, soy sauce, rice vinegar, maple syrup, garlic, gingers, and red pepper flakes. Combine the sauce with the spaghetti and mix thoroughly. Top with green onions. Enjoy hot!

85. **Vegan Chickpea Sweet Potato Curry**: This recipe is a delicious and healthy way to enjoy chickpeas and sweet potatoes. You will need chickpeas, sweet potatoes, onions, garlic, ginger, curry powder, turmeric, cumin, salt, pepper, and coconut milk. In a large frying pan, sauté the onion, garlic, and ginger until fragrant. Mix in curry powder, turmeric, cumin, salt, and pepper. Add chickpeas and sweet potatoes. Cook the sweet potatoes until they become tender. Add coconut milk and mix well. Enjoy warm with rice or naan. enjoy!

86. **Vegan Lentil and Vegetable Stir-Fry**: This recipe is a quick and easy dinner option. You will need lentils, broccoli, bell peppers, onions, garlic, soy sauce, rice vinegar, maple syrup, cornstarch, salt, and pepper. In a large frying pan, sauté the onion and garlic until fragrant. Add broccoli, peppers, and lentils. In a separate bowl, combine soy sauce, rice vinegar, maple syrup, cornstarch, salt, and pepper. Add the sauce to the pot and mix well. Cook until the vegetables are soft. Enjoy with hot rice or noodles. enjoy!

87. **Vegan Mushroom and Lentil Shepherd's Pie**: This recipe is a vegan version of the classic Shepherd's Pie. You'll need potatoes,

vegan butter, almond milk, lentils, vegetable broth, onions, garlic, mushrooms, carrots, peas, thyme, salt, and pepper. Boil the potatoes until soft. Drain and mash with vegan butter and almond milk. In a separate pot, fry onions and garlic until fragrant. Add mushrooms and cook until soft. Add carrots and cook for a few minutes. Combine lentils, vegetable stock, thyme, salt, and pepper. Simmer for 10 minutes. Add peas and cook for another 5 minutes. Preheat oven to 375°F. Layer the lentil mixture in a baking dish and top with the mashed potatoes. Bake for 20 minutes or until golden brown on top. Enjoy hot!

88. **Vegan Tofu and Vegetable Stir-Fry**: This recipe is a quick and easy dinner option. You will need tofu, broccoli, bell pepper, onion, garlic, soy sauce, rice vinegar, maple syrup, cornstarch, salt, and pepper. In a large frying pan, sauté the onion and garlic until fragrant. Add broccoli, bell pepper, and tofu. In a separate bowl, combine soy sauce, rice vinegar, maple syrup, cornstarch, salt, and pepper. Add the sauce to the pot and mix well. Cook until the vegetables are soft. Enjoy with hot rice or noodles. enjoy!

89. **Vegan Butternut Squash Risotto with Leeks and Spinach**: This recipe is a comforting and flavorful vegan dinner option. You will need butternut squash, arborio rice, vegetable broth, green onions, spinach, nutritional yeast, and thyme. In a large pot, sauté the green onions until fragrant. Add the arborio rice and cook for a few minutes. Add vegetable stock and butternut squash. Simmer until the rice is soft. Add spinach, nutritional yeast, and thyme. Mix well. Serve hot.

90. **Vegan Tofu and Vegetable Stir-Fry**: This recipe is a quick and easy dinner option. You will need tofu, broccoli, bell pepper, onion, garlic, soy sauce, rice vinegar, maple syrup, cornstarch, salt, and pepper. In a large frying pan, sauté the onion and garlic until fragrant. Add broccoli, bell pepper, and tofu. In a separate bowl, combine soy sauce, rice vinegar, maple syrup, cornstarch, salt, and pepper. Add the sauce to the pot and mix well. Cook until the vegetables are soft. Enjoy with hot rice or noodles. enjoy!

CHAPTER 9: SNACKS AND DESSERTS

· Healthy and Satisfying Snack and Dessert Recipes

1. **Dark Chocolate Hummus**: This dessert hummus is unexpectedly delicious. It still contains the protein and fiber components of traditional hummus. Try dipping banana or apple slices, pretzels, strawberries, or graham crackers into this sweet chocolate spread.

2. **Caramel Delight Energy Balls**: These easy no-bake cookies are a healthy twist on one of our favorite Girl Scout cookies - chewy caramel, dark chocolate, and toast. It combines roasted coconut with fiber-rich oats instead of sugar and flour. It only takes 15 minutes from start to finish.

3. **Strawberry Chocolate Greek Yogurt Bark**: Slightly sweet Greek yogurt sprinkled with fresh strawberries and chocolate chips can be frozen and crumbled like chocolate bark (but healthier!). This colorful snack or healthy dessert is perfect for both kids and adults. To achieve the creamiest batter possible, use full-fat yogurt.

4. **Apple Pie Energy Balls**: These no-bake apple pie energy balls are easy to assemble and will give your body the energy it needs to get through the afternoon.

5. **Mini Frozen Yogurt Parfaits**: These mini yogurt parfaits are the perfect sweet treat. You can use raspberries, blueberries, or strawberries for these bite-sized parfaits.

6. **Raspberry Coconut Yogurt Bark**: This easy frozen snack or dessert is made using coconut as the yogurt base and topping. The raspberry jam topping and candy-covered chocolate are then

combined to create a sweet and colorful treat.

7. **Homemade oven-dried strawberries**: Homemade oven-dried strawberries, characterized by their rich fruitiness and sweet-sour flavor, can be easily enjoyed by simply heating them in the oven. Enjoy it as is, add it to trail mixes, or use it as a topping for yogurt or ice cream.

8. **Salted Peanut Butter Pretzel Energy Balls**: Easy to make, these energy bites satisfy your sweet and salty cravings and provide the best fuel for your body and brain. Feel free to swap in other nuts, nut butters, or seed butters.

9. **Chocolate Caramel Energy Bars**: These energy bars are the perfect snack to keep you energized throughout the day. Made with dates, almonds and cashews, naturally sweetened with honey and dates.

10. **Strawberry Chocolate Greek Yogurt Bark**: Slightly sweet Greek yogurt sprinkled with fresh strawberries and chocolate chips can be frozen and crumbled like chocolate bark (but healthier!). This colorful snack or healthy dessert is perfect for both kids and adults. To achieve the creamiest batter possible, use full-fat yogurt.

11. **Peanut Butter Banana Oatmeal Cookies**: These cookies are made with just 4 ingredients and are perfect for a quick and healthy snack.

12. **Chocolate Dipped Clementines**: This easy and healthy dessert is perfect for the winter season. The combination of sweet clementine and dark chocolate is sure to satisfy your sweet tooth.

13. **Pumpkin Spice Energy Balls**: These energy balls are perfect for fall and are made with pumpkin puree, oats, and almond butter.

14. **Cinnamon Apple Chips**: These apple chips are the perfect healthy and delicious snack to satisfy your sweet tooth.

15. **Chocolate Covered Strawberry Smoothie**: This smoothie is a

healthy and delicious way to satisfy your sweet tooth. It consists of strawberries, bananas, and cocoa powder.

16. **Chocolate Covered Strawberry Smoothie**: This smoothie is a healthy and delicious way to satisfy your sweet tooth. It consists of strawberries, bananas, and cocoa powder.

17. **Peanut Butter and Jelly Energy Balls**: These energy balls are the perfect healthy and delicious snack to satisfy your sweet tooth. Made with peanut butter, jelly, and oats.

18. **Chocolate Covered Banana Bites**: These banana bites are the perfect healthy and delicious snack to satisfy your sweet tooth. Made with bananas, peanut butter, and dark chocolate.

19. **Pumpkin Pie Energy Balls**: These energy balls are perfect for fall and are made with pumpkin puree, oats, and almond butter.

20. **Chocolate Covered Almonds**: These chocolate covered almonds are the perfect healthy and delicious snack to satisfy your sweet tooth.

21. **Peanut Butter and Jelly Smoothie**: This smoothie is a healthy and delicious way to satisfy your sweet tooth. It consists of peanut butter, jelly, and banana.

22. **Chocolate Covered Almonds**: These chocolate covered almonds are the perfect healthy and delicious snack to satisfy your sweet tooth.

23. **Pumpkin Pie Energy Balls**: These energy balls are perfect for fall and are made with pumpkin puree, oats, and almond butter.

24. **Chocolate Covered Banana Bites**: These banana bites are the perfect healthy and delicious snack to satisfy your sweet tooth. Made with bananas, peanut butter, and dark chocolate.

25. **Peanut Butter and Jelly Energy Balls**: These energy balls are the perfect healthy and delicious snack to satisfy your sweet tooth. Made with peanut butter, jelly, and oats.

26. **Chocolate Covered Strawberry Smoothie**: This smoothie is a healthy and delicious way to satisfy your sweet tooth. It consists of strawberries, bananas, and cocoa powder.

27. **Cinnamon Apple Chips**: These apple chips are the perfect healthy and delicious snack to satisfy your sweet tooth.

28. **Pumpkin Spice Energy Balls**: These energy balls are perfect for fall and are made with pumpkin puree, oats, and almond butter.

29. **Chocolate Dipped Clementines**: This easy and healthy dessert is perfect for the winter season. The combination of sweet clementine and dark chocolate is sure to satisfy your sweet tooth.

30. **Peanut Butter Banana Oatmeal Cookies**: These cookies are made with just 4 ingredients and are perfect for a quick and healthy snack.

31. **Protein Balls**: These protein balls come in 40 flavors and are perfect for a quick and healthy snack.

32. **Smoothies**: Smoothies are a great way to satisfy your sweet tooth while still getting your fruits and vegetables. Add spinach or kale to your smoothie for an extra nutritional boost.

33. **No-Bake Oatmeal Cookies**: These cookies are made without flour or sugar and are perfect for a healthy snack.

34. **Oatmeal Bars**: These oatmeal bars are a great snack to have on hand when you need something quick and healthy.

35. **Cookie Dough Protein Bars**: These protein bars are a great way to satisfy your sweet tooth while still getting some protein.

36. **Protein Cookies**: These cookies are made with protein powder and are perfect for a quick and healthy snack.

37. **Healthy Chocolate Chip Cookies**: Made with almond flour and coconut sugar, these cookies are a healthier version of the classic

chocolate chip cookie.

38. **Acai Smoothie Dessert Bowls**: These acai smoothie bowls are a healthy and delicious way to satisfy your sweet tooth.

39. **Vanilla Avocado Pudding**: This avocado pudding is the perfect healthy and delicious dessert to satisfy your sweet tooth.

40. **Edamame Dark Chocolate Peanut Butter Dip**: This snack is a great way to get some protein while satisfying your sweet tooth.

41. **Roasted Maple Cinnamon Pumpkin**: This roasted pumpkin is the perfect healthy and delicious snack to satisfy your sweet tooth.

42. **Chocolate Covered Almond Butter Banana Bites**: These banana bites are the perfect healthy and delicious snack to satisfy your sweet tooth. Made with bananas, almond butter, and dark chocolate.

43. **Peanut Butter and Jelly Smoothie**: This smoothie is a healthy and delicious way to satisfy your sweet tooth. It consists of peanut butter, jelly, and banana.

44. **Pumpkin Pie Energy Balls**: These energy balls are perfect for fall and are made with pumpkin puree, oats, and almond butter.

45. **Cinnamon Apple Chips**: These apple chips are the perfect healthy and delicious snack to satisfy your sweet tooth.

46. **Chocolate Dipped Clementines**: This easy and healthy dessert is perfect for the winter season. The combination of sweet clementine and dark chocolate is sure to satisfy your sweet tooth.

47. **Peanut Butter Banana Oatmeal Cookies**: These cookies are made with just 4 ingredients and are perfect for a quick and healthy snack.

48. **Strawberry Banana Smoothie**: This smoothie is a healthy and delicious way to satisfy your sweet tooth. It consists of strawberries, bananas, and yogurt.

49. **Chocolate Covered Strawberries**: These chocolate covered strawberries are the perfect healthy and delicious snack to satisfy your sweet tooth.

50. **Peanut Butter and Jelly Energy Balls**: These energy balls are the perfect healthy and delicious snack to satisfy your sweet tooth. Made with peanut butter, jelly, and oats.

51. **Pumpkin Spice Muesli**: This muesli is perfect for fall and is made with pumpkin puree, oats, and spices.

52. **Protein Balls**: These protein balls come in 40 flavors and are perfect for a quick and healthy snack.

53. **Smoothies**: Smoothies are a great way to satisfy your sweet tooth while still getting your fruits and vegetables. Add spinach or kale to your smoothie for an extra nutritional boost.

54. **No-Bake Oatmeal Cookies**: These cookies are made without flour or sugar and are perfect for a healthy snack.

55. **Oatmeal Bars**: These oatmeal bars are a great snack to have on hand when you need something quick and healthy.

56. **Cookie Dough Protein Bars**: These protein bars are a great way to satisfy your sweet tooth while still getting some protein.

57. **Protein Cookies**: These cookies are made with protein powder and are perfect for a quick and healthy snack.

58. **Healthy Chocolate Chip Cookies**: Made with almond flour and coconut sugar, these cookies are a healthier version of the classic chocolate chip cookie.

59. **Acai Smoothie Dessert Bowls**: These acai smoothie bowls are a healthy and delicious way to satisfy your sweet tooth.

60. **Vanilla Avocado Pudding**: This avocado pudding is the perfect healthy and delicious dessert to satisfy your sweet tooth.

61. **Edamame with Dark Chocolate Peanut Butter** Dip: This snack is a great way to get some protein while satisfying your sweet tooth.

62. **Roasted Maple Cinnamon Pumpkin**: This roasted pumpkin is the perfect healthy and delicious snack to satisfy your sweet tooth.

63. Almond Butter and Chocolate Covered Banana Bites: These banana bites are the perfect healthy and delicious snack to satisfy your sweet tooth. Made with bananas, almond butter, and dark chocolate.

64. **Peanut Butter and Jelly Smoothie**: This smoothie is a healthy and delicious way to satisfy your sweet tooth. It consists of peanut butter, jelly, and banana.

65. **Pumpkin Pie Energy Balls**: Perfect for fall, these energy balls are made with pumpkin puree, oats, and almond butter.

66. **Cinnamon Apple Chips**: These apple chips are the perfect healthy and delicious snack to satisfy your sweet tooth.

67. **Chocolate Dipped Clementines**: This easy and healthy dessert is perfect for the winter season. The combination of sweet clementine and dark chocolate is sure to satisfy your sweet tooth.

68. **Peanut Butter Banana Oatmeal Cookies**: Made with just 4 ingredients, these cookies are perfect for a quick and healthy snack.

69. **Loaded Black Bean Dip**: This is a 7 layer black bean dip. Simplified: simply heats up refried beans, season them, and tops them with fresh veggies to create a zesty, textured dip.

70. **Flourless Banana Chocolate Chip Mini Muffins**: Pulsated rolled oats with eggs, banana, brown sugar, and oil create a moist chocolate muffin batter without all-purpose flour. A two-bite muffin with a rich and melty texture. It's slightly sweet and rich. Baked as mini muffins, they're perfect for a snack or morning

snack.

71. **Homemade Multi-Seed Crackers**: Turn leftover brown rice and quinoa from dinner or meal prep into delicious, crunchy crackers with 3 healthy seeds. Adds bagel flavor without the bagel. The whole grains that make up this cracker copycat recipe are rich in fiber, making them a healthy snack that pairs perfectly with hummus and cheese.

72. **Mini Frozen Yogurt Parfait**: This mini yogurt parfait is the perfect sweet treat. You can use raspberries, blueberries, or strawberries for these bite-sized parfaits.

73. **Mini Pebre Peppers**: This version of the chili seasoning Pebre combines peppers, tomatoes, parsley, and cilantro for a fresh flavor.

74. **Mini Peppers Stuffed with Pimiento Cheese**: Make a quick 3-ingredient appetizer by slathering these mini peppers with pimiento cheese.

75. **Loaded Sweet Potato Nacho Fries**: These Loaded Sweet Potato Nacho Fries are a healthier take on the classic nachos. It's loaded with black beans, cheese, salsa, and avocado.

76. **Chocolate Covered Strawberries**: These chocolate covered strawberries are the perfect healthy and delicious snack to satisfy your sweet tooth.

77. **Peanut Butter Jelly Smoothie**: This smoothie is a healthy and delicious way to satisfy your sweet tooth. It consists of peanut butter, jelly, and banana.

78. **Pumpkin Pie Energy Balls**: These energy balls are perfect for fall and are made with pumpkin puree, oats, and almond butter.

79. **Cinnamon Apple Chips**: These apple chips are the perfect healthy and delicious snack to satisfy your sweet tooth.

80. **Chocolate Dipped Clementines**: This easy and healthy dessert is perfect for the winter season. The combination of sweet clementine and dark chocolate is sure to satisfy your sweet tooth.

81. **Peanut Butter Banana Oatmeal Cookies**: Made with just 4 ingredients, these cookies are perfect for a quick and healthy snack.

82. **Loaded Black Bean Dip**: This is a 7 layer black bean dip. Simplified: simply heats up refried beans, season them, and tops them with fresh veggies to create a zesty, textured dip.

83. **Mojito Blueberry Watermelon Salad**: Inspired by the classic Mojito cocktail, this festive and healthy fruit salad takes a special twist with rum, lime, and mint. Optional pimento d'espelette (a sweet and spicy ground pepper from France's Basque region) adds a spiciness that contrasts nicely with the sweet fruit. Look for this spice in specialty stores, well-stocked markets, or online. For a similarly subtle kick, you can use a chili-lime spice blend (like a tagine), or omit the spices altogether. If you prefer a non-alcoholic salad, feel free to omit the rum. With or without rum, this salad is perfect for a summer backyard barbecue.

84. **Flourless Banana Chocolate Mini Muffins**: Pulse rolled oats with eggs, bananas, brown sugar, and oil to create moist chocolate muffin batter without all-purpose flour. A two-bite muffin with a rich and melty texture. Subtly sweet and rich, they are perfect for snacks or morning snacks when baked as mini muffins.

85. **Homemade Multi-Seed Crackers**: Turn leftover brown rice and quinoa from dinner or meal prep into these delicious crunchy crackers with 3 healthy seeds. Adds bagel flavor without the bagel. The whole grains that make up this cracker copycat recipe are rich in fiber, making them a healthy snack that pairs perfectly with hummus and cheese.

86. **Mini Frozen Yogurt Parfaits**: These mini yogurt parfaits are

the perfect sweet treat. You can use raspberries, blueberries, or strawberries for these bite-sized parfaits.

87. **Mini Pebre Peppers**: This version of the chili seasoning Pebre combines bell peppers, tomatoes, parsley, and cilantro for a fresh taste.

88. **Mini Peppers Stuffed with Pimiento Cheese**: Fill these mini peppers with a quick smear of pimiento cheese for an easy 3-ingredient appetizer.

89. **Loaded Sweet Potato Nacho Fries**: These Loaded Sweet Potato Nacho Fries are a healthier take on the classic nachos. It's loaded with black beans, cheese, salsa, and avocado.

90. **Chocolate Covered Strawberries**: These chocolate covered strawberries are the perfect healthy and delicious snack to satisfy your sweet tooth.

91. **Peanut Butter and Jelly Smoothie**: This smoothie is a healthy and delicious way to satisfy your sweet tooth. Consists of peanut butter, jelly and banana

92. **Loaded Black Bean Dip**: This is a 7 layer black bean dip. Simply heats up refried beans, season them, and top them with fresh veggies to create an exciting and textured dip.

93. **Flourless Banana Chocolate Chip Mini Muffins**: Pulsating oat flakes with eggs, banana, brown sugar, and oil create a moist chocolate muffin batter without all-purpose flour. A two-bite muffin with a rich and melty texture. Subtly sweet and rich, they are perfect for snacks or morning snacks when baked as mini muffins.

94. **Homemade Multi-Seed Crackers**: Transform leftover brown rice and quinoa from dinner or meal prep into delicious, crunchy crackers with 3 healthy seeds. Adds bagel flavor without the bagel. The whole grains that make up this cracker copycat recipe are rich in fiber, making them a healthy snack that pairs perfectly with

hummus and cheese.

95. **Mini Frozen Yogurt Parfait**: A mini yogurt parfait that is perfect for sweet sweets. You can use raspberries, blueberries, or strawberries for these bite-sized parfaits.

96. **Mini Bell Pepper Pebre**: This version of the chili condiment pebre combines bell peppers, tomatoes, parsley, and cilantro for a fresh flavor.

97. **Mini Peppers Stuffed with Pimiento Cheese**: Fill these mini peppers with a quick smear of pimiento cheese for an easy 3-ingredient appetizer.

98. **Loaded Sweet Potato Nacho Fries**: These Loaded Sweet Potato Nacho Fries are a healthier take on the classic nachos. It's loaded with black beans, cheese, salsa, and avocado.

99. **Chocolate Covered Strawberries**: These chocolate covered strawberries are the perfect healthy and delicious snack to satisfy your sweet tooth.

100. **Peanut Butter and Jelly Smoothie**: This smoothie is a healthy and delicious way to satisfy your sweet tooth. It consists of peanut butter, jelly, and banana.

101. **Pumpkin Pie Energy Balls**: Perfect for fall, these energy balls are made with pumpkin puree, oats, and almond butter.

102. **Cinnamon Apple Chips**: These apple chips are the perfect healthy and delicious snack to satisfy your sweet tooth.

CHAPTER 10: STAYING MOTIVATED

• Tips for Staying Motivated on a Plant-Based Journey

Here are some tips for staying motivated on a Plant-Based Journey:

1. **Others Get inspired by**: TED - Watching lectures or reading success stories of people who have successfully transitioned to a plant-based diet can help you stay motivated.

2. **Get educated**: Learning about the benefits of a plant-based diet can help you stay motivated. You can learn more by reading books, watching documentaries, and taking online courses.

3. **Plan your meals**: Meal planning helps you stay on track and avoid unhealthy foods. Meal planning apps and websites can make the process easier.

4. **Find support**: Joining a plant-based community or finding plant-based friends can help you stay motivated and accountable.

5. **Start small**: Making small changes to your diet can help you stay motivated and feel less overwhelmed. Start by adding more fruits and vegetables to your diet or trying a new plant-based recipe each week. It can be hard to stay motivated on your plant-based journey, but remember it's worth it for your health and the environment.

Follow these tips and don't be too hard on yourself if you make a mistake. Every small step counts!

• Common challenges and how to overcome them

Switching to a plant-based diet can be difficult, but it's worth it for your health and the environment. Here are some common challenges people face when switching to a plant-based diet and how to overcome them.

1. **Social Pressure**: Social situations can be difficult if you're the only one eating a plant-based diet. You may feel unable to participate in social events or feel judged by others. To overcome this challenge, try to find supportive friends and family to encourage you along the way. You can also bring plant-based dishes to social events or suggest restaurants that offer plant-based options.

2. **Cravings**: When you switch to a plant-based diet, you may experience cravings for foods that were previously your favorite foods. To overcome this challenge, try finding plant-based alternatives to your favorite foods. For example, if you love pizza, try making a plant-based pizza with vegan cheese and lots of vegetables. You can also try new plant-based recipes and find new favorites.

3. **Lack of variety**: Eating the same plant-based meals every day can be boring. To overcome this challenge, try incorporating a variety of fruits, vegetables, grains, and legumes into your diet. You can also experiment with different spices and herbs to add flavor to your meals.

4. **Nutrient deficiencies**: Plant-based diets can be deficient in certain nutrients, such as vitamin B12, iron, and calcium. To overcome this challenge, be sure to eat a variety of nutrient-dense plant foods, including leafy greens, nuts, seeds, and fortified plant milks. You can also take nutritional supplements if needed.

5. **Cost**: Plant-based diets can be expensive, especially if you rely on processed plant-based foods. To overcome this challenge, try eating whole, locally grown, seasonal, plant-based foods. You can also buy in bulk and freeze any leftovers.

6. **Ignorance**: Switching to a plant-based diet can be a daunting task, especially if you're new to plant-based foods. To overcome this challenge, learn about plant-based nutrition and cooking. You can learn more by reading books, watching documentaries, and taking online courses. You can also join plant-based communities and find plant-based friends for support and advice.